HOP TO IT

POETRY ANTHOLOGIES BY VARDELL & WONG

THE POETRY FRIDAY ANTHOLOGY FOR SCIENCE
TEACHER/LIBRARIAN EDITION (K-5)
STUDENT EDITION (THE POETRY OF SCIENCE)

THE POETRY FRIDAY ANTHOLOGY FOR CELEBRATIONS
TEACHER/LIBRARIAN EDITION
STUDENT EDITION

THE POETRY FRIDAY POWER BOOK SERIES
YOU JUST WAIT (TWEENS + TEENS)
HERE WE GO (GRADES 3 + UP)
PET CRAZY (GRADES K-4)

GREAT MORNING! POEMS FOR SCHOOL LEADERS TO READ ALOUD

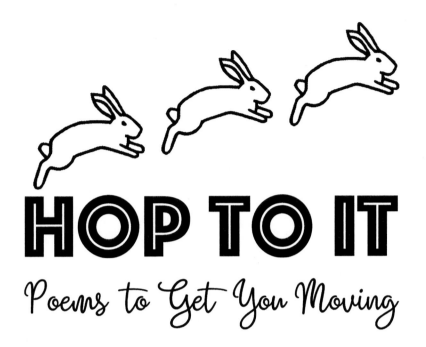

HOP TO IT

Poems to Get You Moving

BY THE CREATORS OF THE POETRY FRIDAY ANTHOLOGY™ SERIES

SYLVIA VARDELL & JANET WONG

ILLUSTRATIONS BY

FRANZI PAETZOLD

Pomelo Books

THIS BOOK IS DEDICATED TO
THE EVERYDAY HEROES

Pomelo Books
4580 Province Line Road
Princeton, NJ 08540
www.PomeloBooks.com
info@PomeloBooks.com

Library of Congress Cataloging-in-Publication Data is available.

ISBN 978-1-937057-29-9

Please visit us:
www.PomeloBooks.com

POETS

Alma Flor Ada	Xelena González	Eric Ode
Kathryn Apel	Joan Bransfield Graham	Linda Sue Park
Rebecca Balcárcel	Paul W. Hankins	Baptiste Paul
Ibtisam Barakat	Janice N. Harrington	Miranda Paul
Michelle Heidenrich Barnes	David L. Harrison	Moe Phillips
Doraine Bennett	Jane Heitman Healy	Jack Prelutsky
Carmen T. Bernier-Grand	Rebekah Hoeft	Deborah Reidy
Robyn Hood Black	Carol-Ann Hoyte	Leslie Ross-Degnan
Susan Blackaby	Ann Ingalls	Shanah Salter
David Bowles	Karen G. Jordan	Darren Sardelli
Jay Brazeau	Jacqueline Jules	Michelle Schaub
Joseph Bruchac	Alan Katz	Robert Schechter
Stephanie Calmenson	Sheila Kerwin	Claire Schlinkert
F. Isabel Campoy	Julie Larios	Laura Shovan
Rose Cappelli	Renée M. LaTulippe	Buffy Silverman
Yangsook Choi	Rebecca Gardyn Levington	Margaret Simon
Lesa Cline-Ransome	Suzy Levinson	Cynthia Leitich Smith
Natalee Creech	Jone Rush MacCulloch	Eileen Spinelli
Ed DeCaria	JoAnn Early Macken	Elizabeth Steinglass
Kristy Dempsey	Marjorie Maddox	Mariahadessa Ekere Tallie
Linda Dryfhout	Kevin Noble Maillard	Holly Thompson
Alice Faye Duncan	Juli Mayer	Linda Kulp Trout
Zetta Elliott	Diane Mayr	Amy Ludwig VanDerwater
Margarita Engle	David McMullin	Sylvia Vardell
Janet Clare Fagal	Sarah Meade	Padma Venkatraman
Carrie Finison	Christy Mihaly	April Halprin Wayland
Nancy Bo Flood	Heidi Mordhorst	Carole Boston Weatherford
Catherine Flynn	Laura Mucha	Tamera Will Wissinger
Marilyn Garcia	Diana Murray	Janet Wong
Charles Ghigna	Lesléa Newman	Helen Kemp Zax

 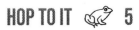

TABLE OF CONTENTS

 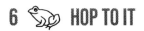

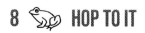

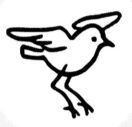

LET'S GET MOVING

Nowadays, we sit a lot. We watch our big screen (and small screen) televisions, play games, check our cell phones, and Zoom online. It can be fun and entertaining and even educational, but it means our bodies are still and we're not getting the exercise we need to keep our bodies healthy and our minds sharp. Some researchers say that young people now average more than seven hours a day with entertainment media. They also say that moving more helps us pay attention better and gives us biological benefits too.

Did you know that the simple act of jumping can give your body more oxygen, improve your balance, strengthen your heart, and increase your energy?

CLAP STAND WAVE JUMP
HOP TWIRL MOVE DANCE

Many of the poems in this book were written for you for just this reason: to read or listen and MOVE. Have you ever chanted a cheer at a ball game that included standing, clapping, or waving? Or joined in a game on a playground with a song or a rhyme that had you jumping, hopping, or twirling? This is how we can combine words and movement through fun rhymes and verses.

In this book, there are poems for doing jumping jacks, dancing in your chair, running in place, moving your feet, wiggling like a worm, and so much more. As experts have said, just like songs are not just sheet music, poetry is not just words. It needs to be read out loud, sung, performed, chanted, pantomimed, dramatized, and brought to life through props and performance and even sign language. Get ready to read and move!

LET'S BE SAFE

We live in a world full of challenges, now more than ever. Many of the poems in this book reflect these times with poems about wearing masks, keeping social distance, worrying about germs and viruses, talking with friends and family via Zoom, and more. Yes, poets write about things we are experiencing right now and help us sort through our complicated feelings during difficult times.

Do you worry about when you can see your friends in person? Or go to the movies? Or hug your grandparents? There are poems about this and more. Reading them can help us feel better and sharing them can help us stay connected.

> The future depends entirely
> on what each of us does every day;
> a movement is only people moving.
>
> **GLORIA STEINEM**

LET'S SPEAK UP

Poets have been protesting problems in society for generations. They use their words to raise questions, to point out issues, to voice complaints, and to rally people to speak up when they see things that are wrong.

There are poems in this book that do this very thing: poems about social activism, consciousness raising, raising your voice, and marching for what's right. Do you see things in the news that bother you? Do you wonder what you can do to make a difference? Many poems in this book will echo these feelings and can help you find your way.

"A journey of a thousand miles begins with **a single step**."
—Lao Tzu

New research found that the average parent spends **five hours and 18 minutes a day worrying** about their kids.

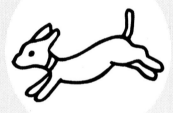

The first protest in the U.S. was the Boston Tea Party in 1773, which eventually led to the American Revolution and the formation of the United States.

Kids can make a difference! Read about one girl who does in *Book Uncle and Me* by Uma Krishnaswami.

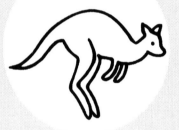
LET'S GET STARTED

When you're feeling stressed or anxious and need help finding a moment of calm . . . look for a poem. Or when you're feeling tired and lethargic and need a jumpstart . . . look for a poem. Or when you're distracted and can't concentrate . . . look for a poem. Or when you just have one minute and need a refreshing break . . . look for a poem. That is what is unique and special about poetry; poems are usually short and don't take long to read, but they can help you relax or get motivated or think clearly or take your mind off your troubles.

In this collection of poems, you'll find examples of all of these things—poems about sitting on the beach, poems about monsters who dance, poems about speaking up for yourself, poems about running and jumping, and so much more.

> In the midst of movement and chaos, keep stillness inside of you.
>
> **DEEPAK CHOPRA**

LET'S READ

In this anthology, every two pages features a pair of poems matched by topic or theme or style. Plus, there are tips for reading the poems and adding movement as you share the poem out loud on every page. You'll also find a related fact, quote, or bit of trivia, and a recommendation of a picture book related to the poem, along with an illustration on the side of each page. And if you need help finding more poetry books about movement, social justice, or health and safety, there are lists of books in the back—along with activities, tips on skill building, and helpful blogs and websites. We hope you'll find escape, information, and inspiration in these pages and share your favorite poems with your friends and family.

TIPS FOR READING A POEM OUT LOUD

Here are some tips to help you read poetry out loud:

- Be sure to **say the title and author** of the poem.
- If you can, **display the words of the poem** for others to see while you read it aloud.
- Be sure to **enunciate each word** distinctly and if you're not sure how to pronounce a word, ask someone or look it up beforehand.
- **Glance at your audience** occasionally.
- For even more fun, **use a portable microphone** or a microphone app.

WHEN TO SHARE POETRY?

1. Share a poem at the beginning of the day, at the end of the day, or during a break.
2. Share a poem during an "announcements" time in school or at a meeting.
3. Share a poem for a special occasion, such as a birthday or anniversary.
4. Share a poem during a meal or snack time.
5. Share a poem while waiting in line.
6. Share a poem **ANY TIME!**

SOCIAL STUDIES AND STEM CONNECTIONS

You'll find fascinating facts and a related picture book on every poem page with a connection to social studies and STEM (science, technology, engineering, and math). You'll learn about the world record for hopping on one foot, why engineers study bluebottle flies, about the youngest Nobel Peace Prize winner, and much more. We hope this will inspire you to learn more on your own—by doing an online search with those keywords or by going to the library to look for books on those subjects.

"Today a **reader**, tomorrow a **leader**."
—Margaret Fuller

Just **20 minutes** of being active improves reading, spelling, math, and memory.

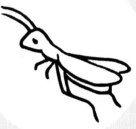

People who take time to **celebrate their successes** are often more optimistic, take better care of themselves, and tend to be less stressed.

Learn about a woman who learned to read at age 116 in **The Oldest Student** by Rita Lorraine Hubbard.

Let those that would
move the world
first move themselves.

SOCRATES

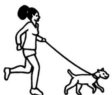

HOP TO IT

by Janet Wong

Burned out?
Tired?
Get rewired.

Hop to it!
Do it.
Reset. Rewake!

S t r e t c h
a minute
then jump back in it.

Hop to it!
Do it.
Take a break!

See if you can read this whole poem out loud while **hopping on one foot**!

What is the Guinness record for the most hops on one foot in 30 seconds? **105 hops!**

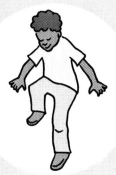

Poets sometimes arrange lines in groups called *stanzas*. These 3-line stanzas are called **tercets**.

Hop, jump, wiggle, and waggle all the way to the library for *Hop, Hop, Jump!* by Lauren Thompson.

Make the motions in this poem while reading it out loud. You can **put a shoe on your hand** for the *foot wave* so you don't fall over!

Rabbits **have a complex language**—ears forward, ears back, or one ear forward and one ear back can mean different things!

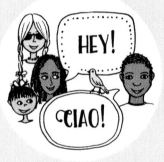

People talk about greetings from *outer* space, and maybe not greetings from *inner* space— but poets love **wordplay**!

Say hello to a whole world full of animals with *Hello Hello* by Brendan Wenzel.

WAYS TO SAY HELLO

by Janet Wong

Foot wave
air bump
jazz hands
heart thump
thumbs up
clap hello
chicken wing elbow
rabbit ears
fish face

I bring you greetings
from inner space

HELLO, FRIENDS

by Sylvia Vardell

I salute hello
like a soldier or a general,
touch my temple
palm down, motion out,
a greeting with respect—

then interlock my index fingers,
curling them together,
left then right, right then left,
showing my friends
our special bond.

Hello, friends!

Try using
sign language for
the words *hello* and
friends as you read aloud.
Hello = a salute motion.
Friends = interlocking
index fingers.

ASL
**(American Sign
Language)** is only one
of several hundred types
of sign language
used throughout
the world.

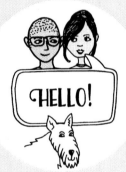

This poem
is an example
of a **how-to poem**.
It gives us specific
directions on how to
do something.

Learn some
ASL together with
someone in your family
with **Hands & Hearts**
by Donna Jo
Napoli.

Walk in place while you read this poem out loud.

Mile comes from the ancient Roman term *mille passus (1,000 paces)*, but most people take more than **2,000 steps to walk a mile.**

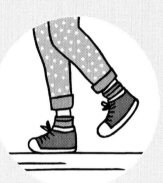

This poem is a great example of a **question poem**. Start a poem with a question of your own!

Imagine standing in the shoes of famous women in **Juno Valentine and the Magical Shoes** by Eva Chen.

WALK ONE MILE

by Baptiste Paul and Miranda Paul

Did you ever stop walking
and take a look down
at the feet that pass by
in your city or town?

Sneakers and flip-flops
and loafers and heels,
sandals and boots—
even footwear with wheels.

These aren't simply shoes
stepping onto a bus.
In them are people
with hearts just like us.

What are their lives like?
How can we know?
First we might start
with a gentle "hello."

WAVE TO ME FROM ACROSS THE STREET!

by Sheila Kerwin

Right now we can't be together.
We can't play side by side.
But I know a place where we can meet:
in our front yards outside!

Neighbors play music. We bounce to the beat.
We shake our hips and tap our feet.
The sun is warm. The flowers smell sweet.
Wave to me from across the street!

I call across, "I miss you!
But we'll be together soon."
I let my hugs float through the air
like a big hot air balloon.

Neighbors play music. We bounce to the beat.
We shake our hips and tap our feet.
The sun is warm. The flowers smell sweet.
Wave to me from across the street!

Get ready to **bounce (hop), shake** your hips, tap your feet, and wave your hands as you read this poem out loud.

Do you like to wave hello? Ed Carlson became famous as The Waver, waving as he walked all over the country for 30 years.

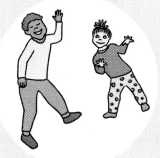

Poets use **simile** to compare things with the words *like* or *as* (*hugs float through the air / like a big hot air balloon*).

Kids find a way to overcome a barrier and let their friendship grow in *The Other Side* by Jacqueline Woodson.

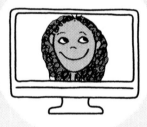

SAME FRIEND, DIFFERENT SIZE

by Marjorie Maddox

You shine in my eye:
small square of smile and wave,
a few inches on my computer.

The teacher calls out your name
from a different small square,
then clicks a key,

so your friendly face
looms large across the screen
and all of us from all our different homes

in bedrooms, basements, kitchens, and dens
are again giggling and guffawing—
the internet crackling with happiness, with joy.

WHAT'S BEHIND MY HEAD?

by Kristy Dempsey

Today I'm in Tahiti,
lounging on the sand.
Tomorrow I'll be up on stage,
rocking with my band.
On Friday, back behind me
there'll be lions on my screen.
Next week, my background vid
will bounce me on a trampoline.
I've got a plan for every day—
my classmates think it's cool.
Each day I'm in a brand new place
when we have online school.

Pantomime each scene in this poem: lie on the beach, rock with a band, act scared of lions, and bounce on a trampoline.

Create your own **virtual backgrounds!** Moyinoluwa Oluwaseun had her own photography business and Instagram account of nearly 20,000 followers by age seven.

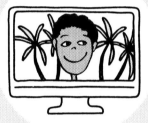

If you can imagine pictures (or even a video) in your mind when you read a poem, it probably has strong **imagery**.

Would you like to make short animated movies? Learn how with *Animation Studio* by Helen Piercy.

**Pretend
you are washing
your hands** while you
read this poem out loud—
it takes about 30 seconds,
as long as we need to
wash our hands to get
rid of germs.

**What does
COVID-19 mean?**
CO = *corona*;
VI = *virus*; and
D = *disease*.
The number 19 refers
to the year of the first
outbreak, 2019.

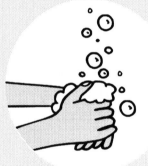

Poets have
different styles
when it comes to
using capital letters.
Sometimes they like to
start each line with
a **capital letter.**

How do
germs spread?
What is a microbe?
Learn about it in
Do Not Lick This Book
by Idan Ben-Barak.

2020

by Jack Prelutsky

We're in a pandemic,
I hardly can stand it.
The mask I must wear
Makes me look like a bandit.
Nothing is normal,
And everything's wrong.
I'm tired of washing
My hands all day long.

I'm tired of keeping
My distance from friends,
And scarcely can wait
Till this misery ends.
The minute we're finished
With COVID-19,
I promise to stop
Being careful and clean.

22 HOP TO IT

MICRO MONSTER

by Laura Shovan

It flies through the air
with the greatest of ease
on a jet stream of goo
when your friend has to sneeze.

This monster's petite,
miniscule, microscopic.
Its devious plans
are quite misanthropic.

From the spikes of its crown
to the plugs on its fingers,
it sticks to the air
where it hovers and lingers.

It flies up your nose.
It is stealthy and quick.
Now you have the virus.
Now you're feeling sick.

Invisible foes
are not easy to conquer,
but it helps, when you sneeze,
if you cover your honker.

This poem has a regular beat and rhythm and you can **sing it** to the tune of *On Top of Old Smoky.* Try it!

Scientists use **electron microscopes** to study viruses; they can magnify a particle up to 10 million times larger than its size.

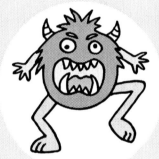

Poets sometimes arrange lines in groups called *stanzas.* These 4-line stanzas are called **quatrains.**

When we're sick, friends can sometimes help us feel better. See **A Sick Day for Amos McGee** by Philip C. Stead.

MASKS FOR ALL!

by Shanah Salter

A mask for me, a mask for you,
to stop the spread of sickness goo.
Whether you are well or sneezy,
wearing a mask is super easy!

Pick one out that fits you right—
snug is good but not too tight.
It can pull on, tie, or hook.
Any mask is a good look!

At school, in any store or street,
in rain or snow or cold or heat,
protecting me, protecting you—
wear a mask, stop germs and flu!

I SMILE WITH MY EYES

by David McMullin

My face may be masked, but I'm not in disguise.
A mask keeps us safe when we all socialize.
I'm showing more feelings than you realize.
How will you know? By the look in my eyes.

If something is shocking? My brows show surprise.
I find a joke funny? My eyes energize.
When someone acts shady, I squint at their lies.
"That's so annoying," my eye roll implies.

As anger grows hotter, my eyes shrink in size.
Say something sad and my tears start to rise.
I'm in on a secret? My wink shows I'm wise.
And when you are near me, I smile with my eyes.

When you read this poem out loud, see if you can **use your eyes and eyebrows** to make the movements in the poem.

Based on research, when we smile **a *true* enjoyment smile**, our eyes narrow and crinkle. With a *fake* smile, the muscles around the eye do not move.

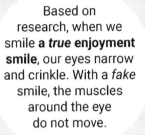

In this **question poem,** the poet asks some questions about himself— and then answers them. Try writing a question poem of your own!

Learn how some animals defend themselves in ***Never Smile at a Monkey*** by Steve Jenkins.

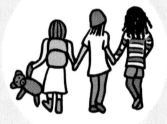

SAY WHEN

by Leslie Ross-Degnan

No school.
No friends.

My life depends

On a virus
So small

I see nothing at all.

Its breath
Is cruel.

It silently rules.

Please leave.
Say when

I can see my friends again.

CHANGING TIMES

by Robert Schechter

The world can change
in the space of a minute,
can rearrange
your life within it,

but the sky never ends—
it will stay there above you,
and your family and friends
will always love you.

This poem
can be read by
two groups—each
group reading one
stanza out loud.
Try it!

**What can
happen in a minute?**
More than five million
pounds of garbage will
be created in the world
and more than
250 babies will
be born.

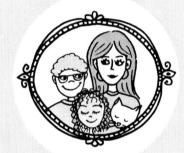

Notice how
the **punctuation**
that the poet used
here allows the poem
to be read as one long
sentence.

There are all
kinds of families!
Let's celebrate many
different families in
***A Family Is a Family
Is a Family***
by Sara O'Leary.

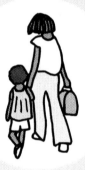

OUR WALK TO SCHOOL

by Rebecca Gardyn Levington

We walk to school each morning.
We take the long way there.
My school is closed, but Mama says:
"It's good to get some air."

We talk about my teachers,
the friends we haven't seen.
We talk about the plans we had
before the quarantine.

We talk about our worries,
our disappointments, too.
We brainstorm new activities—
exciting things to do.

We sometimes walk in silence,
as chipmunks skitter by.
We watch the clouds above us
shifting, drifting in the sky.

When life returns to normal,
to how things used to be,
I hope my mama still makes time
to take these walks with me.

LOOK FOR BIRDS

by Janet Wong

It could be worse.
It *is* worse
somewhere
for someone.

Today will blend into tomorrow.
Tomorrow will become next week.
Everything happening now
will become just one page
in a history book
in a hundred years.

Let's look out the window.
Come, let's look for birds.

Read this poem out loud while **standing near a window** or doorway. What birds can you see?

There are approximately **50 million birders** in the United States (people who look for birds as a hobby).

This poem is an example of **free verse.** It doesn't follow a set of rules, and there isn't a *pattern* of rhyme.

Birds come in many different colors and sizes! See some of them in the book *Birds* by Kevin Henkes.

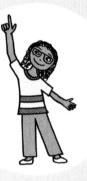

A POEM FOR WHEN THINGS GET A LITTLE TOO SERIOUS

by Heidi Mordhorst

Stretch up and tickle the ceiling—
its giggle is giddy and sweet.

Bend down and tickle the floor—
its chuckle is muddy and deep.

Reach out and tickle the walls—
they snort and whoop and howl.

Reach in and tickle yourself—
giggle and
    chuckle and
        snort and
            whoop
        until you're tickled out!

CARELESSLY HAIRLESS

by Alan Katz

My parents are great.
They're really swell.
I love them both
as you can tell.

I've just one gripe:
I wish they'd stop
playing at-home
barber shop!

It's a hair-don't,
not a hairdo!
I might be bald
when they get through.

Snipping, clipping,
cutting, styling.
Could be weeks
until I'm smiling.

They finish, and
say, "How 'bout that!"
I'm gonna go
put on a hat.

Invite a friend to read **the line in quotation marks** while you read the rest out loud. Pretend you're putting on a hat at the end!

The first drawings of humans (28,000 years ago) show women with long braided hair. The few **early drawings of men show them bald.**

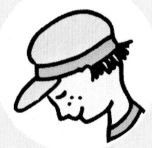

Poets use **wordplay** to twist regular words into clever new words. Next time you get a new *hairdo*, let's hope that it's not a *hair-don't!*

What could be crazier than getting a bad haircut? Giving a monster a haircut: *Even Monsters Need Haircuts* by Matthew McElligott.

Make the **ASL sign for** *no* every time you read *no* in this poem: tap your index finger and middle finger together with your thumb.

In parts of the Southern Hemisphere, **summer vacation** starts in December and lasts through late February or early March.

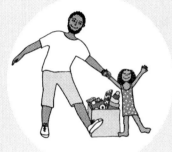

A **list poem** is made up of a list of words or phrases and sometimes uses *repetition* to draw attention to the list.

If you want to camp in the wild or even in your backyard, read **When We Go Camping** by Margriet Ruurs.

STAYCATION

by Michelle Schaub

Our summer vacation
did not go as planned.
No trek to the ocean.
No waves and no sand.
No hike up a mountain.
No ride on a plane.
No lakeside, no cabin.
No tour on a train.
No travel for us
though we love to roam.
But we were together,
safe and at home.
My dad pitched a tent,
and Mom filled the pool.
Our backyard staycation
was still really cool!

THE GREAT INDOORS

by Diana Murray

There's nothing like a camping trip
to make you want to grin.
And with imagination you
can bring the outside in!

First you'll need to pack supplies,
like pillows, books, and toys.
(There might be sleeping bears nearby,
so don't make too much noise.)

Stack some cushions, move some chairs,
spread sheets to make a roof.
Work until you get it right.
Before you know it, POOF!

You'll have yourself a cozy tent
where you can eat some snacks,
wave at parents hiking by,
or kick back and relax!

And who knows what might happen if . . .
you wake a bear that snores!
Adventure never ends when you
explore the Great Indoors.

Try singing **this poem** to the tune of *99 Bottles of Pop*— just for fun!

During the 2020 pandemic, many national parks closed, inspiring some people to **camp indoors.**

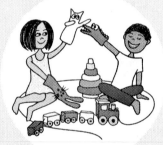

This poem uses **punctuation** (ellipses) in a clever way . . . to create suspense!

Planning a camping trip? This book will help you get ready! *The Camping Trip* by Jennifer K. Mann.

Ask a friend to read this poem out loud while you **pantomime** the many movements of the puppy in this poem.

Bioengineers working to create *super noses* for humans are **studying dogs' noses**. (A dog has 300 million olfactory receptors; we have six million.)

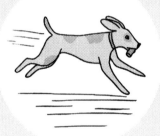

Poets usually put rhyming words at the ends of lines, but sometimes they use **internal rhyme** inside a line (*races/chase/shoelace*).

A dog and a girl shuttle from one home to another in ***Fred Stays with Me!*** by Nancy Coffelt.

FOLLOW YOUR NOSE

by Margarita Engle

My puppy jumps up high
when she smells a butterfly!

She   races   to   chase   my   shoelace . . .

twirls
    in
       circles
  tricked
      by
        swirling
squirrels

and sniffs my hand when I touch a flower,

then curls
beside me, nose in a book
during our peaceful, read-out-loud
once upon a scent
story hour.

A SELF-TRAINED NINJA

by Yangsook Choi

Under the silvery moon
his whiskers glow white
He sharpens his paws on tires
He swats a dozen mosquitoes
He hunkers down in silence

Upon the approaching footsteps
his eyes glimmer orange
He jumps several feet
He strikes the intruder down
He raises his butt in the enemy's face

He is my cat
A self-trained ninja
guarding me while I'm sleeping

Invite a friend to read this poem out loud while you **act like the cat** in the poem—and sharpen paws, swat mosquitoes, and so on.

Using DNA samples from 1,000 cats, a zoologist found that **domestic cats** originated in Mesopotamia more than 100,000 years ago.

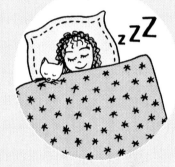

Poets use **metaphor and simile** to compare things, such as *my cat = a ninja*.

Learn the rules for being a *super-awesome* ninja with ***Ninja Bunny*** by Jennifer Gray Olson.

Make the **ASL sign for** *wake* or *awake* as you read this poem: place your hands near your eyes, touch your index finger to your thumb, and open and shut them.

Scientists study the cellular changes that protect squirrels' brains during **hibernation** to develop treatments for human stroke patients.

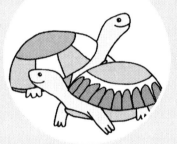

Poets have different styles when it comes to using capital letters. This poem uses no capital letters; it is all in **lower case**.

The world around us is full of morning sounds! Read about them in *What Sound Is Morning?* by Grant Snider.

WAKE THE WORLD

by Holly Thompson

wake the world, the world's awake
turtles are rustling the woodlands awake
trample some leaves, stomp some twigs
explore the floor of the forest awake

wake the world, the world's awake
ducklings are dabbling the pond awake
tip over forward, dunk your face
scoop up some algae for breakfast awake

wake the world, the world's awake
squirrels are gathering nuts awake
scurry then wait, scoop out a hole
bury your stash to eat later awake

wake the world, the world's awake
stretch out your arms to the day awake
breathe in, breathe out
welcome the day with a shake awake

A NEW DAY

by Lesa Cline-Ransome

An alarm chirps
and a family wakes
crawling from beds
and bustling about their nest

Morning showers
revive all

Croaked good mornings
and hasty pecks
begin a day
busy with the
buzzing
brewing
gathering
hauling
sorting
and feeding
that families do
each day
every day
a new day begins

Start your
read aloud of this
poem with an **alarm
clock chirp** (from a
clock, cell phone, or
your own voice).

Birds sing
more in the morning;
scientists call it the
dawn chorus. Do birds
prefer the quiet of
morning because
their songs carry
further?

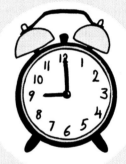

Poets
sometimes use
no punctuation. This
poem has no commas
or periods, but line breaks
and stanza breaks tell
us when to
pause.

Read
about one girl's
morning routine in
My Good Morning
by Kim
Crockett-Corson.

Invite listeners to choose a **favorite activity** from the poem. Skits? Puzzles? Juggling? Baking? They can chime in on those words while you read the rest out loud.

Want to learn another language? Researchers found that **sleeping in between practice** sessions helps people learn another language better.

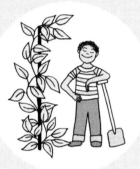

Sometimes poets use **internal rhyme** within a line (*complete/repeat*) in addition to or instead of end rhyme.

Have you ever been afraid to try something difficult? Read about it in ***The Thing Lou Couldn't Do*** by Ashley Spires.

NOW'S YOUR CHANCE

by Karen G. Jordan

Alone and bored? Friends can't play?
Now's your chance to break away
from what you were to who you'll be:
stronger, smarter, easily.
Create a task toward one good goal.
Complete it, repeat it. You're in control!
Grow new muscles. Write some skits.
Finish puzzles. Practice splits.
Learn to juggle. Bake a pie.
Knit a scarf. Give chess a try.
Coding, backbends, violin
are yours to master. You can win
a brand new you, bit by bit.
Small steps work, so stay with it!

#CREATEACHALLENGE

by Kristy Dempsey

Join the trend.
Tag a friend.
Pushup war.
Dance floor.
Foot shake.
Egg break.
Pass the ball!
Chair. Wall.
Match Dad's moves.
Catch Mom's grooves.
Make it spiral.
Go viral!

Plan your read aloud of this poem with a friend. **Take turns reading** the lines in an alternating pattern and then both read the final line together.

Some **challenges** are charitable: the Ice Bucket Challenge raised $115 million for research in the fight against ALS.

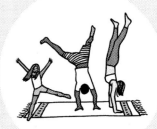

A **list poem** is made up of a list of words or phrases; in this poem, each line describes a different social media challenge.

A friendly little challenge can get us doing fun things. See what happens in *The Pink Refrigerator* by Tim Egan!

Read this poem out loud and invite others to join in on the names of the **days of the week** (*Monday, Wednesday,* and *Saturday*).

When does a new day start? For thousands of years, astronomers counted a day from noon to noon, but now we count it from midnight to midnight.

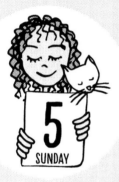

Repetition is a technique poets love to use. You can repeat single words, parts of lines, whole lines, or even just the pattern of a sentence.

Do different days have special meanings for you? They do in ***Monday Is One Day*** by Arthur A. Levine.

CAN I PLEASE HAVE A CALENDAR?

by Moe Phillips

Can I please have a calendar?
The kind you hang on the wall.
It's the only way I'll ever know
what day it is at all.

Monday is just like Wednesday.
Has Saturday gone away?
Feels like every day's the same.
I can't tell school from play.

If I could have a calendar,
the kind you hang on the wall,
I'd know again what day it is
and look forward to them all.

STUCK

by Eileen Spinelli

I'm stuck in my room. Almost over the flu.
And sure—I have plenty of things to do:
video games, iPad and iPod,
texting with Tara and Carmen and Todd,
comics, crayons, cards and TV,
a kit to make a bonsai tree.
You'd think that all this stuff of mine
would keep me occupied just fine.
Yet—life is feeling such a bore.
Then—
my little sister comes by my door
with her toy radio on the floor.
Music plays and off she goes
twirling round on tippy-toes,
dancing with a silly wiggle.
I can't help myself—I giggle.
"You dance too!" She sends a grin.
I give a shrug and then give in.
This dancing is good medicine!

Invite a friend to read the words in quotation marks while you read the rest out loud. Pretend you're **dancing** as you read the last two lines.

Dance reduces stress, increases levels of the *feel-good* hormone *serotonin*, and helps improve memory.

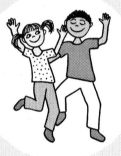

What do you do for fun at home? Let the four *list lines* in this list poem (*video games / texting / comics / a kit*) inspire you to write your own poem!

What to do if you're sick? Try to keep your germs to yourself. Read this to learn what *not* to do: *Sick Simon* by Dan Krall.

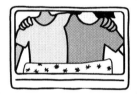
ZOOM DOOM

by Helen Kemp Zax

Higgledy piggledy,
Grandma and Grandpapa
Zoom with our family at
night from their beds,

where they're confused by the
camera placement and—
oops!—accidentally
cut off their heads.

LOCKDOWN FREEDOM

by Claire Schlinkert

The people went home. They shut up their shops.
The city was still and the animals came.
The mountain goats munched upon manicured hedges
and capered with joy through their reclaimed terrain.

The stoats and the weasels went off on vacation,
a "once-in-a-lifetime"-billed sightseeing tour.
And everywhere, buzzards and badgers and warblers
and otters and orcas set off to explore.

The sheep flocked to playgrounds to ride on the roundabouts.
No social distancing. No one could fuss,
for we were locked down, like some back-to-front zoo where
the animals gathered to goggle at *us*.

Invite people to **say the names of the animals** while you read this poem out loud (*mountain goats, stoats, weasels, buzzards,* and so on).

People make wild animals nervous: when scientists set up speakers and played recordings of people's voices, mountain lions became jittery.

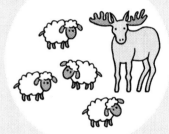

This poem contains many examples of **alliteration,** such as *shut/shops, mountain/munched/ manicured,* and so on.

Would it be fun to have zoo animals visiting your house? Find out in *The Way to the Zoo* by John Burningham.

Walk like a pigeon while you read or hear this poem: bob your head forward as you move around. Pigeons do this to track their surroundings.

Pigeons can **find their way back to their nests** from as far as 1300 miles away, which is why they have been used throughout history as messengers.

When the speaker in a poem is non-human and normally unable to talk, we can say that the poem is in the **voice of the mask.**

Pigeons might be amazing, but do we want them to drive? See *Don't Let the Pigeon Drive the Bus* by Mo Willems.

PIGEON PANACHE

by Carrie Finison

We pigeons don't just walk the street
that throbs with people, trucks, and trains.
We strut our stuff. We feel the beat.
The city pulses in our veins.

Alone, in pairs, or feathered flocks,
we swagger up the thoroughfares.
We promenade down city blocks,
and swarm in plazas, parks, and squares.

Weaving, bobbing, pecking crumbs,
staring down the passing cars,
dodging when a stroller comes—
these streets are ours and we're the stars!

RABBIT DANCE

by Joseph Bruchac

Over the meadow
a full moon is shining
almost as bright as the sun.

It is the time when
the rabbits all gather
after the day's light is done.

Making a circle
they dance in the moonlight
hopping and stomping their feet,

hearing the music
that's kept in their hearts
moving to that ancient beat.

I've never seen them
dancing and dancing
but I know that it is so.

I've seen their footprints
all in a circle
there in the late winter snow.

Listeners can do a *binky*, **a happy rabbit dance,** while you read this poem aloud: jumping up, twisting, and turning their heads back and forth.

Some rabbits binky more than others. Some just do a half-binky, called a head flick or ear flick, while others turn 180 degrees mid-air.

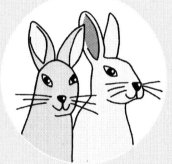

When a poem makes us very aware of our senses (sight, hearing, smell, taste, or touch), it has strong **imagery.**

Rabbits star in many folktales, such as this fun retelling of an Iroquois tale: *Rabbit's Snow Dance* by Joseph Bruchac and James Bruchac.

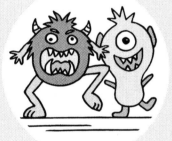

MONSTERS DON'T DANCE

by Ann Ingalls

Monsters don't dance, we stomp.
Monsters don't prance, we clomp.
Thumping and clumping all over the place,
With a howl and a growl and a scowl on each face.
Jumping around as we bippity-bop.
Pumping our arms as we hippity-hop.
Striding and gliding, we romp, and we clomp.
Monsters don't dance, we stomp!

LET'S DANCE

by Linda Dryfhout

I wiggle my toes
and tap my feet.
I shift my legs
and feel the beat.

I swivel my hips
from left to right.
I shimmy my shoulders
that feel tight.

I swing my arms
to and fro.
I shake my hands
up high, down low.

I bob my head.
I'm in the groove.
Come on, let's dance.
Join me. Let's move!

Make all the motions included in the poem (wiggling toes, tapping feet, and so on) as you read it out loud.

Square dancing is the official state dance of more than 30 states; some others are the Charleston, polka, clogging, and Texas Two-Step.

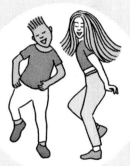

If you follow the steps in this **how-to poem**, you'll find yourself dancing by the end!

We can learn about dances from all over the world in the book *Let's Dance* by Valerie Bolling.

Invite half your listeners to **tap their feet** and the other half to **slide side to side** with arms out wide, while you read the poem out loud.

Dance Marathon events all over the world have raised millions of dollars to help children with cancer.

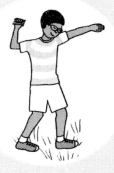

In this example of 4-line stanzas (**quatrains**), the rhyme pattern is different than what we've seen in other quatrains in this book. Hooray for variety!

Dancing in a special event can take lots of time and work, as we see in the powwow preparations in *Jingle Dancer* by Cynthia Leitich Smith.

FEEL THE BEAT

by Stephanie Calmenson

We tap, tap, tap
our feet.
Feel the beat—
it's real sweet.

We hold our arms
out wide
as we slide—
side to side.

We'll sell tickets
to our show.
Money we
raise will go—

to feed kids who
need to eat.
So take a seat—
feel the beat!

BE THE BEAT!

by Buffy Silverman

You're a musician.
Your desk is the drum.
Wiggle your fingers, your hands, your thumbs.

Tap a rhythm—
Tippity Tap. Tippity Tap.
Tap. Tap. Tap.

Snap a rhythm—
Snap. Snap. Snap.
Snap. Snap. Snap.

Clap a rhythm—
CLAP-clap-clap-clap. CLAP-clap-clap-clap.
CLAP. CLAP. CLAP.

Wiggle your fingers, your hands, your thumbs.
You're a musician.
Your desk is the drum!

Use your desk or a table as your poetry prop and **tap, snap, and clap** (when it occurs in the poem) as you read this poem out loud.

Hand drums are played all around the world, such as the pandeiro (Brazil), tabla (India), taiko (Japan), and cajon (Peru).

Poets like to use **onomatopoeia**—words that sound like the sounds they make (*tippity tap, snap, clap*).

Read about a girl who played drums—and changed history—in the book ***Drum Dream Girl*** by Margarita Engle.

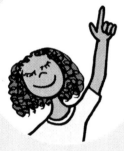

THIS ONE

by Paul W. Hankins

This
one
finger
right
here
can
push
a button
called
"home"
and make something
happen. In an instant:
I'm searching; I'm swiping.
I'm selecting and I'm saving.
But, with this one finger I can
also conduct an invisible band
heard only to my ear as I sweep
the sweet sounds through space.

MUSIC IN MY TOWN

by David Bowles

There's music in my town,
everywhere I go—
we shop and work and learn,
carried on its flow.
Oldies at the barber shop,
cumbias in the store,
songs at church and school,
through every open door!
My face can't help but smile,
my feet just have to move—
life is best just like this,
living to a groove.

Ask a friend
to **play or sing a song**
in the background as
you read this poem out
loud—ending with a
few dance
moves!

Do your
**feet *just have to
move*** to music? When
certain music is played,
the part of our brains
called the cerebellum
makes us move
our legs.

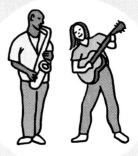

This poem
is presented in
one single stanza,
though the poem could
have been split into three
stanzas. Choices make
it fun to write
and revise!

Many places
come alive with
music and dance,
especially at night!
See them samba in
Cats' Night Out
by Caroline
Stutson.

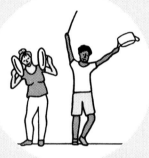

CITY SONG

by Marilyn Garcia

Every night at seven o'clock
we climb the stairs right to the top.
We see the city's empty streets
and break its silence with our BEATS!
AND BANGS! AND CLANGS!
AND CHEERS! AND CLAPS!
Our SHOUTS! AND STOMPS!
AND FINGER SNAPS!

To show we know how much they give
so
WE CAN BREATHE
so
WE CAN LIVE.

Note: During the COVID pandemic in Spring 2020,
many people went outside and made noise to thank
health care workers at 7pm each evening.

HEARTBEAT

by Jane Heitman Healy

Thuh THUMP, thuh THUMP,
Heartbeat, fist bump,
Thuh THUMP, high five,
Heart beat. I'm alive!
Thuh THUMP, I soar,
Heartbeat, I roar!
Thuh THUMP, I jump!
Heartbeats, blood pumps.
Thuh THUMP, beat fast,
Thuh THUMP, beat strong,
Thuh THUMP, Thuh THUMP
Is my heart's song.

Place your open palm on your chest over your heart and **pat it rhythmically** while you read this poem out loud.

While a human heartbeat is usually between **50-100 beats per minute**, a hamster's heart beats 450 times per minute.

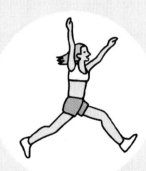

Repetition is one of the best tools that a poet can use to make music in a poem—and it can also add to the meaning of a poem.

Explore the music and power of our heartbeats in this story about whales: *Heartbeat* by Evan Turk.

As you read this poem out loud, invite your listeners to **say a key word** (*tiger* or another word you choose) after the lines that end in a period.

Earworm is the term for a song that gets stuck in your head. According to one psychologist, 90% of people experience an earworm at least once a week.

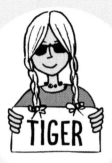

This **free verse** poem doesn't follow a set of rules—and even though there is some rhyme in it, there isn't a *pattern* of rhyme.

Do you have favorite words? Start a collection of them, as in **The Word Collector** by Peter H. Reynolds.

YOUR SONG

by Doraine Bennett

Say a favorite word—
tiger, red, stars, ice cream.
Whisper it like a question.
Tiger? Tiger?
Again and again.
Answer with your word.
Big and bold.
Feel how it sounds
as it moves up and down
or down and up
or around and around.
Say it softly like a lullaby.
Stretch it out slow and long.
Sing it to yourself,
like it's a song.
Sing your word.
Sing high or low
until you find the note
that's all yours.
Let it roll off your tongue.
Let it settle in strong.
Who are you?
Say your word.
Sing it like a song
you know by heart.

EXERCISING MY VOICE

by April Halprin Wayland

I can yawn, hum,
wiggle my tongue,
blow through a straw,
I can drop my jaw.

I can trill my lips
like a motor in a lake,
I can sing eeeee ooooo,
I can hissss like a snake.

I'm getting ready
in the thick of this chatter
to tell the world
that MY VOICE MATTERS!

When you read this poem out loud, **make the motion** or sound described in the poem after you say each line.

This poem was inspired by the **nine best vocal warm-ups** for singers, according to SchoolofRock.com, from yawning to humming to hissing.

Many words that we use for animal sounds—such as *hiss*—are examples of **onomatopoeia.** They sound like the things they describe.

Young voices can make a difference! See *No Voice Too Small* edited by Lindsay H. Metcalf, Keila V. Dawson, and Jeanette Bradley.

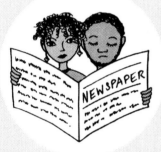

YOU CAN DO IT RIGHT NOW

by Janet Wong

You can shout at a march.
You can quietly pray.
You can read the news
and share it today.
You can send the mayor
of your town a note.
You can make a sign
that tells people to vote.
You can talk to your family.
You can listen to friends.

There are different ways
to reach the same ends,
to fight injustice,
to show that you care.

You can do it right now,
from anywhere.

STAND UP

by Christy Mihaly

Be a friend when someone's hurting.
Give a smile or helping hand.
Don't be shy about asserting
what is right: just take a stand.
Stand up!

If you want to make things better,
think of things that you can do.
Make a call or send a letter.
Illustrate your point of view.
          Stand up!

In a tizzy, feeling nervous?
Know your rights and learn your laws.
Join a march or day of service.
Find some friends to join your cause.
          STAND UP!

Don't just sit there on the sidelines
when you see there's work to do.
If you think we need new guidelines,
write them up—it's up to you!

                    STAND UP!

Sit as you read this poem out loud, then **stand up** when you read *Stand up!* and challenge three other people to stand up with each new *Stand up!* line.

Who is the youngest person to win the **Nobel Peace Prize?** Malala Yousafzai, at age 17.

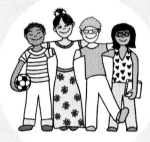

Poets might **capitalize words or put them in *italics*** to draw attention to them and to suggest that we say these words more powerfully.

When we see bullying or other wrongs, we can follow the lead of the kids in ***Get Up, Stand Up*** by Bob Marley.

When you read this poem aloud, you have to **march in place!**

At age nine, Audrey Hendricks participated in **the Children's Crusade** and was the youngest person ever to be arrested for protesting.

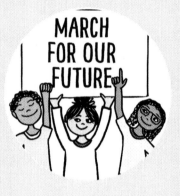

This poem has a distinctive and regular **rhythm.** Clap loudly when you hear a stressed beat, and clap softly when you hear an unstressed beat.

Thousands of children marched for justice in the Birmingham Children's Crusade of 1963. **Let the Children March** by Monica Clark-Robinson tells their story.

MARCH!

by Suzy Levinson

We march for a future that's brighter,
for justice, for freedom, for choice.
We march because we have the power
to fight for what's right with our voice.
Equality! Peace! Education!
Nothing can stand in our way!
We march for a better tomorrow
that starts with a better today.

WALKING

by Diane Mayr

Get out the paint and cardboard.
Add words to make a sign.
Gather with a community
whose purposes intertwine.

Changing a culture's not easy.
You start by changing minds.
Be active in a community
that practices being kind.

Walk for peace and justice.
Leave no one behind.
You're part of a community
that wants us all to shine.

Read this poem aloud with friends, with each person **standing up** when a new line begins and joining in together.

Protest art can include a simple poster you make yourself, a famous painting by Picasso, or the street graffiti of the artist Banksy.

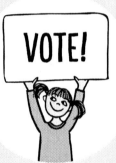

This is a **poem of address**, where the poet is speaking to someone. Poems of address often use the word *you* (*You start by changing minds*).

Imagine a place where everyone is loved and appreciated, then read about the school in **All Are Welcome** by Alexandra Penfold.

As you read this poem aloud, **gesture to each body part** as it is mentioned in the poem (*muscles, arms, heart, mind, eyes,* and *feet*).

The heart is the hardest-working muscle of the approximately 600 muscles in your body.

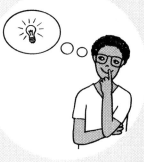

Poets have their own styles when it comes to **punctuation and capitalization**. See how this poem uses no commas, periods, or capital letters.

Let's celebrate our minds, muscles, hearts, and all of ourselves in *I Am Every Good Thing* by Derrick Barnes.

EVERYDAY USE

by Zetta Elliott

our muscles
grow strong with
everyday use
strong arms can offer
a tender embrace
a heart that is brave
can soften with compassion
a clever mind can
find time to daydream
sharp eyes can see
both sides of a problem
and the fastest feet
can slow to march
the long road
to justice

THE LOUDEST OF HANDS

by Kevin Noble Maillard

Raise your fist in the air
like you really do care.
Extend your arm
to the sky
and make your
movement
talk.

Listen to the
subtle speech and rhythm
of your own body—

Your small gesture
is physical,
the meaning colossal.

Elevate your fist
to connect with the heavens above
and shine.

Raise your fist in the air as you read this poem out loud, then cup your ear to listen, then raise your fist again for the final stanza.

Many people view a raised fist as a **symbol of unity** because the fingers of an open hand can be hurt more easily than fingers that are united in a fist.

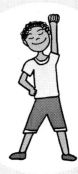

This **free verse** poem doesn't follow a set of rules—and even though there is some rhyme in it, there isn't a *pattern* of rhyme.

Have you ever raised your hands or fist in joy and celebration? See *Hands Up!* by Breanna J. McDaniel.

HANDS SAY, "GREAT JOB!"

by Linda Kulp Trout

Thumbs up
Fingers snap

Jazz hands
Knuckles tap

High five
Clap, clap, clap—

Pat yourself
On the back!

HAND WASHING SONG

by Robert Schechter

Sometimes I chuckle
when scrubbing a knuckle.

Sometimes I hum
while scrubbing a thumb.

I have no qualms
getting suds on my palms.

And I never fail
to clean under each nail.

I can't resist
washing up to my wrist!

I'm careful! I linger
on each dirty finger.

Germs have no hope
thanks to water and soap!

Pantomime all the parts of the **hand washing process** as you read this poem out loud.

Soap and water alone don't kill germs; they work together by removing germs from your hands, if you wash well enough (for at least 20-30 seconds).

This poem is arranged in **rhyming couplets**, 2-line stanzas made up of lines that rhyme with each other.

Need some basic reminders about washing your hands? Find them in *Germs Are Not for Sharing* by Elizabeth Verdick.

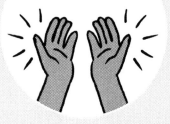

A POEM FOR TIRED HANDS

by Natalee Creech

Place your palms upon your desk
and stretch your fingers wide.
Bend your wrists from left to right—
keep moving side to side.
Lift your fingers one by one.
Squeeze tight and make two fists.
Stretch your hands above your head,
then rock and roll your wrists.
Hands in front, and shake your fingers—
let them all fly free.
Walk your fingers down your legs
and rest them on your knees.

CAPTAIN TOES

by Tamera Will Wissinger

Toes left!

Toes right!

Toes Up Down Up!

Twisty — Twitchy toes—

like a playing pup.

Toes scrunch!

Toes s t r e t c h!

Whenever I choose.

I'm *CAPTAIN TOES*

inside my shoes!

With your shoes off (or on), **move your toes** as you follow the words of this toe-twitching poem.

Two *polydactyl* cats (polydactyl = six or more toes on each paw) are tied for the Guinness World Record for **greatest number of toes: 28**!

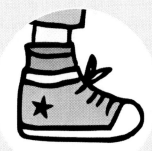

When poets use a **simile** to compare two things, they usually include the words *like* or *as* (*Twisty — Twitchy toes — / like a playing pup*).

See dogs wiggle, jiggle, and even hula hoop in *Wiggle* by Doreen Cronin.

Move your wrists, hands, ankles, and feet and **clap and stamp** as you read this poem out loud.

A human baby has between 275–300 bones, but adults have only 206; several **bones fuse** into single bones as we grow older.

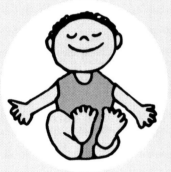

Sometimes poets use **capital letters** for emphasis, to draw attention to certain words.

How do our skeletons compare to other animals'? Find out in *Bones* by Steve Jenkins.

BONES & MATH

by Joan Bransfield Graham

Two hundred and six bones
make your body
complete—
54 in wrists and hands,
52 in ankles and feet.
When you clap
and stamp
in both of
these zones—
SURPRISE!—
you're *moving*
OVER HALF
of your bones!

FIT AS A FIDGET!

by Kathryn Apel

Fidget feet are pretty neat—
they rarely stop or slow.
They keep my teachers on their toes
and help me go-go-go!

They're not like dogs that know the trick
of how to sit and stay.
My fidget feet cannot stand still—
they twitch and tap all day.

When other kids complain of pins
and needles, I don't peep.
I guarantee, my fidget feet
will never go to sleep!

While you read this poem out loud, **bounce back and forth** from one foot to the other on your own *fidget feet.*

Some people use fidget spinners, stress balls, or even smooth stones as **fidget objects** to calm down and stay focused.

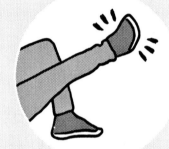

Finding **alliteration** can be a fun game. Can you find some?

fidget/feet;
stop/slow; teachers/toes;
sit/stay; stand/still;
twitch/tap; kids/complain

If your feet are happy being *fidget feet*, celebrate them by reading *Dancing Feet!* by Lindsey Craig.

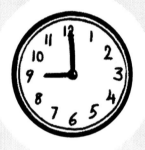

WAITING

by Amy Ludwig VanDerwater

How long
will this take?
I'm waiting
waiting
in
a
line.
I look around.
I tap my foot.
I hum a tune.
I almost whine.
It's hard to learn
it's not my turn.
I slouch.
I stand up straight.
I wait.
I wait.
I wait.
I wait some more.
Wait.
What am I
waiting for?

WIGGLE YOUR EARS!

by Jay Brazeau

It helps if you concentrate.
Calm yourself.
Stare.
Fix your mind.
Grip your chair.

Are you ready?
Go!

Twiddle 'em!
Fiddle 'em!
Flail 'em with flair!

Did they jiggle?
A little?
No?
Don't despair.
If your ears won't wiggle—
try wriggling your hair!

Can you **concentrate and wiggle your ears** while you read this poem out loud? Give it a try!

Scientists have found that approximately 15 percent of humans can **wiggle their ears.**

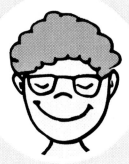

The lines in this poem vary quite a bit in length. Do you see how these **alignment** choices make certain words stand out?

We can celebrate all kinds of ears with the book ***Do Your Ears Hang Low?*** by Jenny Cooper (based on the popular song).

Flossing
cleans out things
between your teeth, and
some people think of
mental floss as changing
your thinking to clear
useless info.

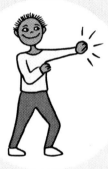

Poets
sometimes
arrange lines in
groups called *stanzas*.
These 3-line stanzas
are called
tercets.

Learn about
hip-hop, cha-cha, and
additional dances in
Feel the Beat
by Marilyn Singer.

MENTAL FLOSS

by Catherine Flynn

My brain is tumbling,
my thoughts are jumbling.
I need to take a break!

Out of my seat,
up on my feet.
I'll give my hips a shake.

Swing my arms, fists clenched tight,
front and back, left then right,
like wipers in the rain.

This mental floss
will shine and gloss
and energize my brain!

CHAIR DANCING

by Xelena González

Boogie your bottom.
Wiggle in your chair.
Wave your hands all around
Like you just don't care!

Let those hands do the clapping,
Toes do the tapping,
And mix it all up
With some sassy snapping.

The dance floor is waiting,
Still empty right now . . .
You can be the brave first!
Want to know how?

Mind off. Body on.
Give yourself a good dare.
And until you're set to go,
Warm up in your chair.

When you read this poem out loud, you should be **sitting in a chair** as you do all the motions and gestures in the poem.

The Rollettes, a team of **wheelchair dancers**, travel the world and believe that *Dance is dance, whether you're walking or rolling.*

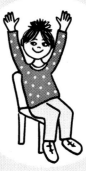

This poem is centered, an **alignment** choice. It works well with the subject of this poem, keeping us sitting in the middle of our chairs!

Celebrate the joy of dancing with this story inspired by a wheelchair-bound dancer: *I Will Dance* by Nancy Bo Flood.

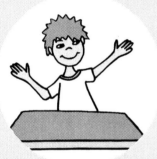

DESKERCISE

by Juli Mayer

Raise your hands up in the air.
Twist your body in your chair.
Touch your nose and blink your eyes.
This is how we deskercise!

Move your feet and march in place.
Pose a sad, then happy face.
Flap your arms, it's time to fly.
This is how we deskercise!

Roll your head and finger snap.
Shrug your shoulders, clap, clap, clap.
Drum your fingers, look surprised.
This is how we deskercise!

MY DESK IS A RACE CAR

by Charles Ghigna

My desk is a race car.
That's what I pretend.
I lean left and right
Around each bend.

My desk is a bike.
I'm riding to town.
My feet on the pedals
Go round and round.

My desk is a jet.
I steer to the sky.
I pass through the clouds
And soar way up high!

Sit at a desk to read this poem out loud and prepare to **lean, pedal, and steer** as you read.

Old airplane parts are often recycled or *upcycled* into new things, such as tables, desks, and chairs.

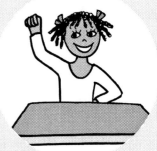

The poet uses **repetition** here not just to repeat the phrase *My desk is*, but also to repeat the structure of each stanza.

If you like the idea of a desk as a race car or bike or jet, how about hover desks? Look for *If I Built a School* by Chris Van Dusen.

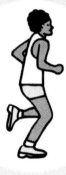

WARMUP CHANT

by Ed DeCaria

We're running in place!
We're running in place!
A hurry-to-nowhere-and-back-again-chase!

We're running in place!
We're running in place!
No finish in sight to this unending race!

We're running in place!
We're running in place!
We're panting, we're sweating, we're red in the face!

We're running in place!
We're running in place!
How long can we keep up this punishing pace???

We're running in place!
We're running in place!
We're running still running STILL RUNNING IN PLACE!

*(Repeat until your coach/teacher finally lets you stop
running in place.)*

CLICK! CLACK! JUMPING JACK!

by Eric Ode

Click! Clack!
Jumping Jack!
Up and down,
out and back.
Arms go up,
legs go wide.
Legs snap tight,
arms at your side.
Back and forth,
one to ten.
Out and back
and out again.
Up and down.
You've got the knack.
Click! Clack!
Jumping Jack!

Poems can be exercise! Read this poem out loud while doing **jumping jacks.**

It is believed that **jumping jacks** were invented by General John Pershing as a training drill at West Point in the early 20th century.

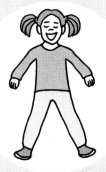

This poem is presented in one single **stanza**, though the poem could easily have been split into four stanzas. Choices make it fun to write and revise!

Busy bodies bounce and stretch and run to the library to look for fitness books like *The Busy Body Book* by Lizzy Rockwell.

As you read this poem out loud, try making the **tae kwon do punching motions** described in the poem.

Tae kwon do students **start with a white belt** and, as they improve, move to yellow, orange, green, blue, purple, brown, red, red and black, and then black belts.

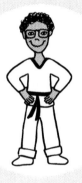

When poets use a **simile** to compare two things, they usually include the words *like* or *as* (*I rise like dust*).

Martial arts skills can be useful, as we see in *Ninja Red Riding Hood* by Corey Rosen Schwartz.

TAE KWON DO PUNCH

by Yangsook Choi

I rise like dust
to strike a blow against my fear.

Hana!   Straight punch!
Dul!   Round punch!
Set!   Side punch!
Net!   Rear punch!

I work my way up the ranks.
I'm a black-belt of hope.

Note: The words *hana, dul, set,* and *net* mean *one, two, three,* and *four* in Korean.

THE P.E. INSTRUCTOR TEACHES A CLASS OF YOUNG SNAKES

by Linda Sue Park

Come and gather—
do not dither!
No more blather,
hiss, or blither!

Group one—hither!
Group two—thither!

All together—

Ready?

SLITHER!

Add gestures
while you read this
poem out loud—a
gesture for *come*, *one*,
two, *together*, and
slither.

Experts
recommend that
owners of snakes give
their pets at least **fifteen
minutes of exercise**
per week, such as
supervised
swimming.

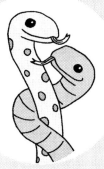

Poets love
playing with words.
Searching for rhymes
can lead a poet to use
unusual words that they
might never have
thought of
using!

If you find
snakes fascinating,
you will love the book
Snakes
by Nic Bishop
with its many photos
of snakes in
action.

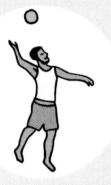

BALL CHANT

by Carol-Ann Hoyte

Woot, woot! Come one, come all!
Everybody grab a ball!

Volley, volley, volleyball!
What do you do with a volleyball?
> *I bump the ball with my arms outstretched*
> *and fingers intertwined.*

Basket, basket, basketball!
What do you do with a basketball?
> *I hoist the ball above my head and*
> *shoot it in the hoop.*

Tennis, tennis, tennis ball!
What do you do with a tennis ball?
> *I whack the ball and lob it high*
> *and deep onto the court.*

Golf, golf, golf ball!
What do you do with a golf ball?
> *I swing my club and putt the ball*
> *along the rolling green.*

A ball is round and never ends.
But this is the end of our chant, my friends.

ALL TIED, BASES LOADED

by Michelle Heidenrich Barnes

The crowd is hyped.
They do the wave.
Next batter up is looking brave.

But I'm brave too.
I stare him down
from here, atop my pitcher's mound.

He swings—a miss!
Strike one! Crowd cheers.
The roar is music to my ears.

Fast ball. He swings—
and hits a foul.
Clapping, stomping, home fans howl!

Can I do this
one more time?
He wants a hit—pride's on the line.

I throw a curve,
then start to doubt.
He swings—
　　　(can't watch)

　　　　　Strike three! YOU'RE OUT!

Invite your listeners to **be like a crowd at a baseball game** while you read the poem out loud like a sportscaster.

Pitcher Jim Abbott, born without a right hand, won an Olympic gold medal for baseball and played on a professional team for ten seasons.

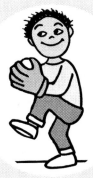

A **narrative poem** tells a story. The story in this poem is told from a *first-person* point of view (*I stare him down*), but usually a narrative poem is in *third person*.

Read about Mamie Johnson, the first female pitcher to play on a professional men's baseball team: *Mamie on the Mound* by Leah Henderson.

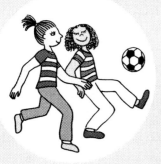

FOOTWORK FOR SOCCER PLAYERS STUCK INSIDE

(for use with a regular, mini, soft, or imaginary ball)
by Elizabeth Steinglass

tip it
tap it
back and forth

trap it
stop it
on the floor

lift it
juggle it
foot to foot

send it
higher
thigh to thigh

higher
still
use your head

count
your touches
as you go

VIRTUAL HOOPS

by Rebekah Hoeft

My friend from school felt far away.
We used to hang out every day.
We felt alone till we got smart
and now we play though we're apart.
We go outside, both grab a ball,
connect our tablets with a call.
He waves and smiles, we laugh and talk.
We mark Around the World with chalk.
And then we play. He shoots.
A miss. I shoot and miss. He hoots
and then he makes three in a row.
We air high-five. Oops, power's low.
We have to stop, but that's okay—
my friend seems not so far away.

Find a friend to read this poem out loud with you— taking turns to **read lines in alternating order** back and forth.

Some of the **first public basketball teams** in the U.S. had nine players throwing a soccer ball into peach baskets nailed to the balcony in a gym.

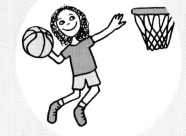

This is an example of a **lyrical poem**, usually a serious poem where poets tell us in first person (I/me/my/mine) how they are feeling.

Learn about basketball's greatest players in *B Is for Baller* by James Littlejohn.

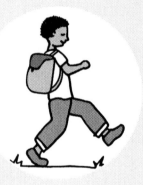

TRAIL READY

by Robyn Hood Black

We're going on a hike today!
I'll get my backpack ready.
Jacket, flashlight, extra socks—
can you hold it steady?
Trail mix, thermos, bug spray, hat,
notebook, pencils, this and that.

Binoculars and whistle
dangle from my neck.
Blue bandanna, walking stick.
Map and compass? Check.

Through the leafy canopies
to fields, where sun is brighter—
Next time (huff) we hike (huff puff),
I'll pack a little lighter.

RISE UP TALL

by JoAnn Early Macken

Pretend you are an acorn.
Crouch down small.
Then grow into an oak tree.
Rise up tall.

Your feet are roots, so plant them
in the ground.
Your arms are branches. Reach up.
Wave them round.

Make room for birds and squirrels.
Stretch out wide.
The wind blows. Lean a little,
side to side.

Stand tall. Imagine growing
all year long.
Pretend you are an oak tree.
You are strong!

Invite listeners to **act out this poem** as you read it out loud—crouching down, growing, reaching, stretching, and leaning together.

There are 600 species of oaks in the world, with 90 in North America. **The national tree** of many countries, including the United States, is an oak.

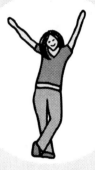

This is a **poem of address**, where the poet is speaking to someone. Poems of address often use the word *you* (*You are strong!*).

Redwoods regularly grow to be more than 200 feet tall. Read about them in *Redwoods* by Jason Chin.

Coach your listeners to **breathe in deeply** as you read the first line, then exhale slowly with the second line, continuing in an alternating pattern.

Trees have been found to be linked underground through **fungal networks** that scientists call the *wood wide web*.

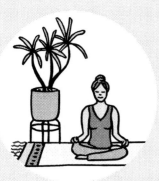

Poets use **metaphor** to compare things (*I am a tree*). This poem features an *extended metaphor*; the idea of the speaker as a tree is used all the way through.

Have you ever pretended to be a tree? Try it—but first read *The Happiest Tree* by Uma Krishnaswami.

ZEN TREE

by Margaret Simon

I am a tree.
A tree is what I want to be.
I spread my branches wide.
I stand tall.
I reach my roots into deep earth.
I grow and grow and grow.
And at the end of the day,
when the sun falls down
and sprinkles orange over all my leaves,
I wrap myself in a holding hug.

ON A BEACH

by Suzy Levinson

Picture it: you're on a beach.
Below you, sand. Above you, sky.
Listen to the crashing waves.
Listen to the seagulls cry.
Palm trees whisper overhead,
swaying in the gentle breeze.
Sunlight hugs you, head to toe.
Close your eyes, be still, and breathe.
Take a breath, long and deep.
Let it out, soft and slow.
Feel your body growing heavy,
sinking in the sand below.
Focus on the sand and sun.
Feel the salty ocean spray.
As you inhale, as you exhale,
all your worries wash away.

Encourage your listeners to close their eyes and **picture the scene** in this poem as you read it out loud slowly, with a pause at the end of each line.

Scientists say that listening to the **sound of ocean waves** can help you relax and strengthen your brain.

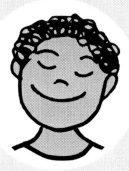

This **how-to poem** gives us specific directions, line-by-line, to help us calm ourselves by slowing our breathing and imagining being on a beach.

There are so many ways to enjoy your time at a beach. Visit one in *Beach* by Elisha Cooper.

Get ready
to move your arms
and legs in **swimming
motions** as you read
this poem
out loud.

Tom Gregory,
the **youngest person
to swim the English
Channel** (at age 11),
trained by taking
cold baths and
showers for over
eight months.

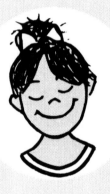

Two of
the lines in this
poem are only one
word long. Do you see
how these interesting
alignment choices
draw your eyes to
certain words?

Swimming
lessons can be
fun—and funny—in
1, 2, 3, Jump!
by Lisl H. Detlefsen.

CLEAR, COOL BLUE

by Jacqueline Jules

Lift your arm in a circle
over your head
and imagine your hand
diving
into the water,
gliding
past your waist
while your other arm
rises over your head
and plunges, too,
into clear, cool blue.

Imagine your feet
fluttering side by side,
swiftly moving through
the clear, cool blue.

Imagine your mind
so calm, surprising you,
in clear, cool blue.

ME AND THE BEACH CREATURES

by Susan Blackaby

I could play at the beach all day!
As the tide rolls in.

Sea lions bask and bark and clap,
As the tide rolls in.

Seagulls squawk and hop and flap,
As the tide rolls in.

Crabs scoot sideways across the beach,
As the tide rolls in.

Lobsters snap their big claw feet,
As the tide rolls in.

I could play at the beach all day!
As the tide rolls in.

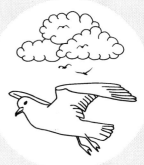

Ask two friends to join you in reading this poem—one to be Sato Dog, one to be Little Blue Crab—while everyone says, *On your mark, get set, go!*

Most **wild animals compete** for food, territory, and mates—all important for survival—but scientists aren't sure they *enjoy* winning like many humans do.

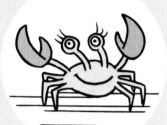

A **narrative poem** tells a story. The story in this poem is told from a *third-person* point of view by a *narrator*.

Read about another Little Crab in ***Don't Worry, Little Crab*** by Chris Haughton.

SATO DOG AND LITTLE BLUE CRAB

by Carmen T. Bernier-Grand

Sato Dog and Little Blue Crab
stand on the starting line.
No dog catcher has been able to catch Sato.
For sure Little Blue Crab won't win.

"On your mark, get set, go!"
Little Blue Crab takes off after Sato Dog.

Sato is almost to the finish.
He turns around to look back.
His tail is almost touching the finish line.
"I don't see Little Blue Crab,"
he growls. "I'm the winner!"
Little Blue Crab climbs down Sato's tail.
Her largest pincer touches the finish line.
"I am the winner!"

YOU CAN'T CATCH ME

by David L. Harrison

Watch me crawl
better than an ant.
Watch me zoom
quicker than a bee.
Watch me leap
higher than a deer.
Ha-ha-ha,
you can't catch me.

Watch me squirm
better than a worm.
Watch me hop
better than a flea.
Watch me scratch
better than a dog.
Ha-ha-ha,
you can't catch me.

Challenge listeners to **sign** *watch me* as it occurs in the poem while you read aloud. ASL = point to yourself with your first two fingers at eye level.

Peregrine falcons are the **fastest animals**, diving at over 200 miles per hour—but the fastest *land* animal is the cheetah, able to run about 70 miles per hour.

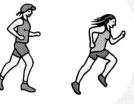

The heavy use of **repetition** in this poem makes it sound like a playground chant or a song.

How quick are bees? African American scientist Charles Henry Turner studied bees and more. Learn about him in *Buzzing with Questions* by Janice N. Harrington.

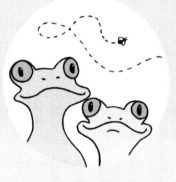

CAN YOU WIGGLE LIKE A WORM?

by Rose Cappelli

Can you wiggle, wiggle, wiggle
Like a worm, worm, worm?
Can you jiggle, jiggle, jiggle
As you squirm?

Can you paddle, paddle, paddle
Like a dog, dog, dog?
Can you hop, hop, hop
Like a frog?

Can you climb, climb, climb
Like a cat, cat, cat?
Can you flap, flap, flap
Like a bat?

Wiggle, jiggle,
Paddle, hop,
Climb, flap,
STOP!

 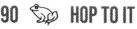

ANYONE HOME?

by Nancy Bo Flood

Walk with a friend
Or all alone
Turn over a stone
Anyone home?
Grubs, bugs, and
One tiny worm
Wiggle
Squirm

Grab a partner and read this poem out loud together—taking turns alternating lines.

Velvet worms (or *onychophora*) live hidden under rocks and in rotting logs—and have changed very little in the last 500 million years.

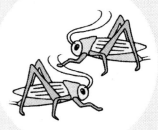

Poets have different styles of capitalization. Sometimes they like to start each line with a **capital letter.**

Can a stone be a kitchen? It is many things in *A Stone Sat Still* by Brendan Wenzel.

As you read this poem out loud, encourage your listeners to **move with you**—arms, body, and feet—in each stanza.

Approximately 65 percent of our **drinking water** comes from rivers. The world's rivers also make it possible for people to wash and bathe.

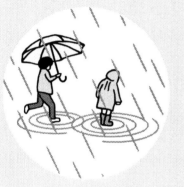

Poets use **simile** to compare things with the words *like* or *as* (arms . . . *like branches*; body . . . *like water*).

Imagine how it feels to float for hundreds of miles down a river in a canoe when you read *River* by Elisha Cooper.

IN NATURE

by F. Isabel Campoy

Wind, wind
arms moving free
like branches in a tree.

River, river
body dancing free
like water in a stream.

Rain, rain
feet playing free
in a puddle in my street.

EN LA NATURALEZA

por F. Isabel Campoy

Viento, viento
brazos al aire en libertad,
ramas de árbol en la ciudad.

Río, río
baila el cuerpo en libertad
corriente de agua en la vecindad.

Lluvia, lluvia
pies danzando en libertad
en un charco en mi comunidad.

AT THE EYE

by Padma Venkatraman

I am lightning. I rip across the sky.
I am a storm, chasing clouds up high.
I am howling wind, whipping at trees.
I am thundering rain on trembling leaves.

As you read aloud, listeners **make rain, storm, and thunder noises** with their hands: rubbing palms together, snapping fingers, and patting laps repeatedly—slowly, then quickly.

The *eye of the storm* is the small area of calm in the middle of a hurricane; the *eyewall* of winds around the eye is the worst part of the storm.

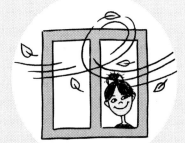

Poets use **metaphor** to compare things implicitly, without the words *like* or *as* (*I am lightning*).

Prepare for a tornado, forest fire, or hurricane by reading *I Am the Storm* by Jane Yolen and Heidi E.Y. Stemple.

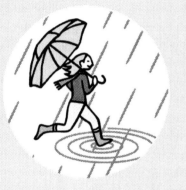

ANY WEATHER

by Rebecca Balcárcel

Thunder stomps
      its rumbly feet,
        flattening clouds to gray gauze.
Frost tiptoes,
      grass to branch,
        leaving glitter footsteps.
Rain races,
      speeding down
        to dirt, head first.
Sun stretches
      glowing arms,
        continent to continent.
I shimmer
      all day long
        in (watch me!) any weather.

 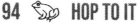

UMBRELLA

by Jone Rush MacCulloch

On
rain days

Umbrella
opens, protects
as we puddle jump

Soon
sunshine—

Raise an umbrella as you read this poem out loud, or use the ASL sign: stack two fists on top of each other, then raise your top fist like you're opening an umbrella.

The U.S. Patent Office has received more than 3000 plans for **redesigning umbrellas,** including attempts to create a flying umbrella.

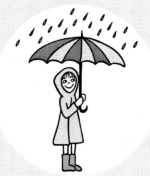

This poem is an example of **free verse**. It doesn't follow a set of rules, and there isn't a *pattern* of rhyme.

Imagine an umbrella that gives everyone shelter, then read **_The Big Umbrella_** by Amy June Bates and Juniper Bates.

Encourage listeners to **look at a color** of their clothing and then join in on the line and movement that corresponds to that color as you read the poem out loud.

Like scientists today, Isaac Newton observed **six colors in the rainbow,** but he was pressured to name seven to match the musical scale—and added indigo.

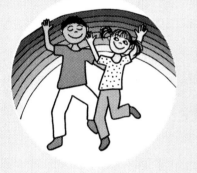

A **list poem** is made up of a list of words or phrases. In this poem, each line (except the last line) lists a color.

Learn about Edwin Binney, the inventor of Crayola crayons, in **The Crayon Man** by Natascha Biebow.

RAINBOW DANCE

by Sarah Meade

Red-red-red: run in place.
Orange: stretch up high.
Yellow: spin around, and then—
Green: flip-flap to fly!
Blue-blue-blue: leap three times.
Indigo: stomp your feet.
Violet: clap and snap and tap.
Rainbow dance—complete!

RAINDROPS AND WORDS

by Ibtisam Barakat

Sometimes I lean on a tree
to rest my feet and my heart.

I point my toes to the sky and dream.
As my toes wiggle in the wind

they watch clouds cross the sky
skating like schoolchildren.

Sometimes a cloud looks down,
slows down,

and becomes curious about me
like I am curious about clouds.

We begin a conversation
of raindrops and words.

Lean
on a wall
(or a tree) as you
read this poem
out loud.

Clouds look
lightweight, but
the average fluffy
cumulus cloud weighs
more than a million
pounds.

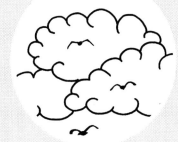

This poem
is arranged in
couplets, 2-line stanzas;
these are unrhymed,
but couplets usually
rhyme.

Have you ever
looked at clouds and
seen . . . sheep?
Imagine away with
It Looked Like Spilt Milk
by Charles Shaw.

This poem
is full of activities!
Invite your listeners to
give a **thumbs up for
their favorite activities**
as you read the poem
out loud.

Psychologists
suggest that we
can **boost our immune
systems** when we write
with the purpose of
understanding and
learning from our
emotions.

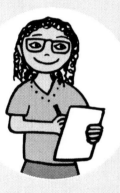

The phrase
I can is repeated
six times in this poem.
Try writing a poem using
repetition, repeating
I can or some
favorite words.

How can
we find courage?
This book will help:
When You Are Brave
by Pat Zietlow Miller.

WHEN I FEEL SCARED

by Janet Wong

When I feel scared and
don't know what to say,
I can draw. I can write.
I can read. I can play.

I can make up a story,
draw a dragon or fox,
build a world out of words,
or Legos or blocks.

Everything in my world
will be good, will be fair.
And with pencil and paper
I can always go there.

THE ARTIST

by Mariahadessa Ekere Tallie

When I don't have words
but I want to talk,
I use my crayons
or sidewalk chalk.

I draw the things
I feel and see
so they don't stay locked
inside of me.

Draw in the air as you read this poem out loud. Can your listeners guess what you have drawn?

In 2015, more than 3000 people in Greeley, Colorado used chalk to draw for 3.5 miles; the **chalk art** set a world record.

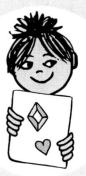

Poets sometimes arrange lines in groups called *stanzas*. These 4-line stanzas are called **quatrains.**

Are there special things that make you feel more creative? Read *Emma's Rug* by Allen Say.

Invite others in the room to chime in on their **favorite holidays.** If they like all the holidays, they can say them all!

Poet Lesléa Newman says, *Read, read, read! Read every book you can get your hands on. And* **write, write, write!**

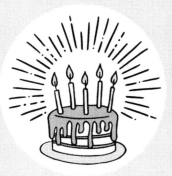

This **list poem** lists fourteen different holidays. Can you write a list poem with some of your favorite holidays?

Most writers agree: you need to revise, revise, and REVISE! Read about it in *You Have to Write* by Janet Wong.

"DO YOU EVEN WRITE ON YOUR BIRTHDAY?"

by Lesléa Newman

I write on Thanksgiving,
on Halloween, too,
on Chanukah, Kwanzaa,
and Christmas, don't you?

On Mother's Day, Father's Day,
Fourth of July,
I put pen to paper
and watch the words fly.

On Easter, on Passover,
Valentine's Day,
my poetry tells me
what I've got to say.

St. Patrick's Day, April Fools,
and New Year's Eve,
like magic I pull
stanzas out of my sleeve.

And yes, on my birthday,
whatever my age,
I blow out the candles
and start a new page.

CUMPLEAÑOS IMAGINARIO

por Alma Flor Ada

Los cumpleaños son alegres
si se saben disfrutar
y no me importa la fecha
para poderlo planear.

Dibujo a los invitados
en pedazos de papel
Juan, Enrique, Marta, Julia,
y mi buen primo Daniel.

Escribo notas amables
pues les quiero agradecer
los simpáticos regalos
que me quisieron hacer.

Lo único que necesito
para poder celebrar
es un pastel delicioso
que me prepare mamá.

Si ellos no pueden comerlo
porque sólo son papel
yo seré muy generoso
¡no dejaré rastro de él!

A MAKE-BELIEVE BIRTHDAY

by Alma Flor Ada

Any time is perfect
for a holiday,
just plan to have fun
your very own way!

I draw my guests
Marta, Enrique, and Bob.
And three more friends:
Silvia, Janet, and Rob.

I write thank you notes
so that they will see
how much I enjoy
the gifts they gave me.

The only thing missing
on this happy occasion:
one of Mom's cakes
for the celebration.

If my paper friends
cannot eat the cake,
I'll be very thoughtful
and leave a clean plate.

Invite your listeners to join you in saying the **names in this poem** as you read the rest of the poem out loud.

Translators often try to match the sound and spirit of a poem rather than the exact meaning, even choosing different names for musical effect.

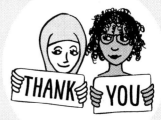

In many **quatrains,** the second and fourth lines rhyme, as they do in both the Spanish and English versions of this poem.

Celebrate yourself every day! Get inspired with *The Birthday Book* by Todd Parr.

Invite listeners to read the **words in parentheses** while you read the rest of the poem out loud.

According to some reports, over 90% of the households in the United States buy **bananas** at least once a month.

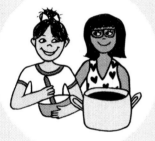

A how-to poem gives specific directions on how to do something, much like a recipe in a cookbook. This **recipe poem** will help you make your own delicious cake!

Follow another recipe, this time for Native American fry bread, after reading *Fry Bread* by Kevin Noble Maillard.

BANANA CAKE BEAT

by Renée M. LaTulippe

On rainy days, I love to bake!
Here's what I need to make a cake:

- three bananas (gone brown-black)
- a couple eggs (to tap and crack)
- a stick of butter (soft and fluffy)
- baking soda (makes cakes puffy)
- light brown sugar (adds some sweet)
- vanilla (goes with any treat!)
- two cups flour (give or take)
- cinnamon (but just one shake)—
   (Oopsy-daisy! Small mistake!)

Mix it with a bit of lovin'—
now it's ready for the oven!

I hope you, too, will try to bake.
It's easy as a piece of cake!

I STOOD ON THE CEILING

by Darren Sardelli

I stood on the ceiling for seventeen minutes.
I walked up a lavender wall.
I danced on a doughnut with strawberry filling
and touched every light in the hall.
I sat on a mushroom and anchovy pizza.
I spun and dove into a pie.
I love being me! Yes, I'm happy and free!
It's incredible being a fly!

Challenge listeners to **guess what creature** this poem describes. Then read it out loud and let them join in on the last word, *fly!*

Mechanical engineers study bluebottle flies landing upside-down in a flight chamber to help create drones that can fly the same way.

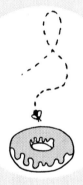

Mask poems are often written in the voice of an animal, but sometimes poets pretend to speak from the point of view of an inanimate object.

Can you imagine a fly as a friend? If the answer is no, maybe you just haven't met the right fly. See *Hi! Fly Guy* by Tedd Arnold.

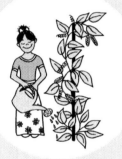

TONIGHT

by Julie Larios

Tonight out the window I see my tomatoes,
my radishes, snap peas, and baby potatoes.
Tomorrow I'll water, tomorrow I'll weed,
tomorrow I'll do what my vegetables need.
But tonight while I'm sleeping the moon will shine down
on those veggies asleep in their beds in the ground.

NO MATTER WHAT

by Laura Mucha

You pick, pack,
stack, prepare,
keep shelves
and bellies full.
You nourish us,
you grow, you share.
No matter what,
you're always there.

Thank you.

Note: Even in a crisis, food workers are on
the job, sometimes risking their own lives
to produce food and keep grocery stores
and markets stocked with essential goods
for the rest of us.

Read this
poem out loud
and invite listeners
to **stand and chime in**
on the final line,
Thank you.

The average
grocery store has
approximately **40,000
items** for you to buy.
(Thank you again,
food workers!)

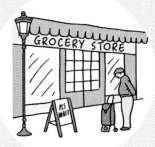

This **poem
of address** uses
the word *you* all
throughout the poem
(*You pick; You nourish;
you grow; you share*).

Hooray
for all the people
who grow, gather,
and deliver our food!
Celebrate them with
Before We Eat
by Pat Brisson.

Encourage your listeners to close their eyes and **imagine the moment** in this poem as you read it out loud slowly.

Researchers have found that the human brain can recognize and remember about **5,000 faces.**

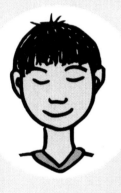

This short poem is a **tanka**, a Japanese poetic form that usually has five lines and syllable counts of 5-7-5-7-7. Tanka often focus on human relationships.

Sometimes small things touch us most—a homemade gift or even just someone who will listen. Read *The Rabbit Listened* by Cori Doerrfeld.

WHEN I CLOSE MY EYES

by Janet Wong

when I close my eyes
and quiet my mind I can
see us together—
each summer you always saved
the first tomato for me

ONE

by Janice N. Harrington

When you're the only one,
the tall one, the short one,
the one with glasses,
the one with braces,

when you're the only one
who came from there,
the only one with frizzy hair,

when you're the only one
and feel like there's a big fat sign
hanging above your head or
an alarm calling:
      the only one!
      the only one!
      the only one!

Remember—
there are lots of only ones.
One + one + one + one
means you're part of a crowd.
You fit right in.
Just look for all the other only ones
and you'll have lots of friends.

Invite seven **people** to join you in reading this poem out loud, saying one of *the only one* lines. Everyone else can raise an index finger for the word *one*.

Since ancient times, there has been a link between solitude and enlightenment; **time spent alone** allows more mental focus.

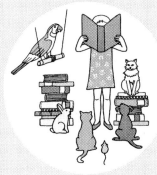

This **free verse** poem doesn't follow a set of rules—and even though there is some rhyme in it, there isn't a *pattern* of rhyme.

How can we share our stories? How can we make friends? You'll see in ***The Day You Begin*** by Jacqueline Woodson.

Your listeners can **point to each body part** mentioned in the poem as you read it out loud—*eyes, hands, ears, feet, legs, heart, brain.*

Read about **young people who are changing the world** like Greta Thunberg, Malala Yousafzai, Marley Dias, Jahkil Jackson, and others.

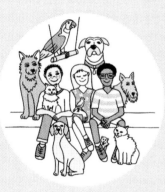

Are you a kid? In this **poem of address**, the poet is speaking to you. *YOU can light up the world!*

There are so many things that make us special. We can all see ourselves in *I Am Enough* by Grace Byers.

CALLING ALL KIDS

by Janet Clare Fagal

Inside of you:
dreams,
ideas.
Wildness, maybe?

Eyes that show
your hands what to draw,
music that only you may hear.
Feet that tap a rhythm.
Legs that like to skate or run.
A tender heart
full of caring.
Words that want to find
their place on a page,
a brain that seeks
to learn, to know.

Like the sky lit
by fireworks,
you are brilliant.
You can light up the world.

SOUL MAGIC

by Alice Faye Duncan

I read books and
Make dreams happen.
I open my mouth and the
Whole world listens.

The people talk my talk.
They dance my dance.
I am SOUL MAGIC like
Harriet, Martin, and Coretta.

I am my Daddy's sky.
I am my Mama's star.
I have no beginning.
My soul is ancient.

Find a friend to read this poem out loud with you, each person reading two lines, taking turns **back and forth.**

You may know **Harriet Tubman, Martin Luther King, Jr., and Coretta Scott King,** but what about Alvin Ailey, Katherine Johnson, and others? Read about them!

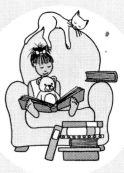

Poets have different styles when it comes to using capitalization. Sometimes they like to start each line with a **capital letter.**

Black is history and culture and celebration and more in ***Black Is a Rainbow Color*** by Angela Joy.

Stand up **and move** in the way the poem describes while you read it out loud, then sit down when you read the last line.

Do **capes** help superheroes aerodynamically? Engineering experts say no, it's the opposite: they generate a drag force and would flutter and slow them down.

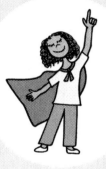

This poem uses **punctuation** (ellipses) for dramatic effect, creating a sense of suspense . . . and making us curious to read what comes next!

Superheroes can be useful around the house, as we see in *Traction Man Is Here* by Mini Grey.

SUPERHERO

by Cynthia Leitich Smith

Up, up, and . . . no way!
I hop, bounce, leap . . .
but my feet land
thud, thud, thud
too quickly.
Up, up, and . . . my way!
Head back, arms raised . . .
flying high
in my imagination.

REACH!

by Rebecca Balcárcel

I can reach the light switch.
I can reach the sink.
On tippy toes, I catch a cup
And fill it up to drink.

I can reach for people
Who need my helpful hands.
With careful reach, I stroke a cat
Who purrs and understands.

I can reach for bravery.
I can reach for dreams.
I stretch so tall, I tap a star
And twirl inside its beams.

Encourage your listeners to **make a *reach up* motion** every time they hear the word *reach* as you read this poem out loud.

According to psychologists, **people who volunteer** have better health and are happier than people who do not volunteer.

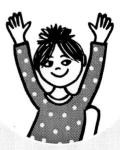

This poem contains several examples of **alliteration** (*tippy toes, catch/cup, helpful hands, tall/tap/twirl*).

Do people around you inspire you to do good things? Then you'll see yourself in *I Can Do It Too!* by Karen Baicker.

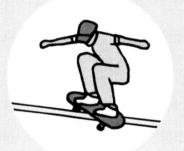

WHEN I MOVE

by Carole Boston Weatherford

When I swim, I become a fish.
When I jump, I become a wish.
When I run, I become the heat.
When I dance, I become the beat.
When I bike, I become the wind.
When I flip, I become the spin.
When I lift, I become the strength.
When I stretch, I become the length.
When I grind, I'm beyond extreme.
When I climb, I behold my dream.
When I move, I'm a force so free
I feel the planet move with me.

PEP TALK FOR A COUCH POTATO

by Eileen Spinelli

If a bee can dance, if a lamb can leap,
if a shark can swim even in its sleep,
if a goose can waddle, if a duck can splash,
if a squirrel can scamper, if a cat can dash,
if a frog can hop . . . and a kangaroo . . .
then you can get a move on too!

Invite nine people to join you, each one moving like one of the animals in the poem, as you sit, read out loud, and then move, too.

Old TVs contain cathode-ray tubes (CRTs). *Tubes* sounds like *tubers* (such as potatoes), so **couch potato** became a way to describe people watching a lot of TV.

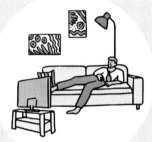

Here's another stellar example of how **rhyme, repetition, and rhythm** can work together to create music in a poem.

What happens when the power goes out? If you're a couch potato, prepare with *The Couch Potato* by Jory John.

Lead your audience in **moving any which way** while you read this poem out loud; everyone will freeze, stop, and stand as you finish the poem.

Tag was played in ancient Greece. In freeze tag, tagged players cannot move until teammates unfreeze them with a touch.

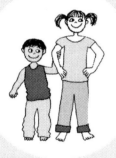

Poets sometimes **capitalize** words to draw attention to them. Here, the way the lines are broken also highlights the capitalized words.

Play ball, skate, and do cartwheels with *Tag Your Dreams* by Jacqueline Jules—but when it's time to stop playing . . . FREEZE!

FREEZE

by Deborah Reidy

MOVE
any which way you want.
MOVE
every which way you can.
But when you hear
FREEZE!
if you please,
STOP moving.
Just
STAND.

EXTRA, EXTRA!

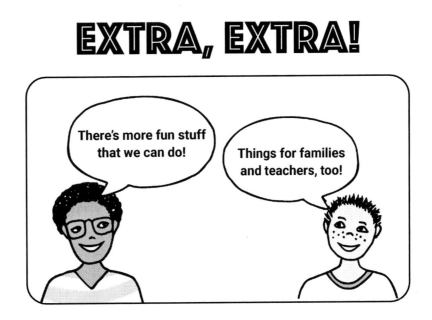

POEM HUNT

Can you find one poem in this book for each of these clues?
Hunt with a friend, if you like!

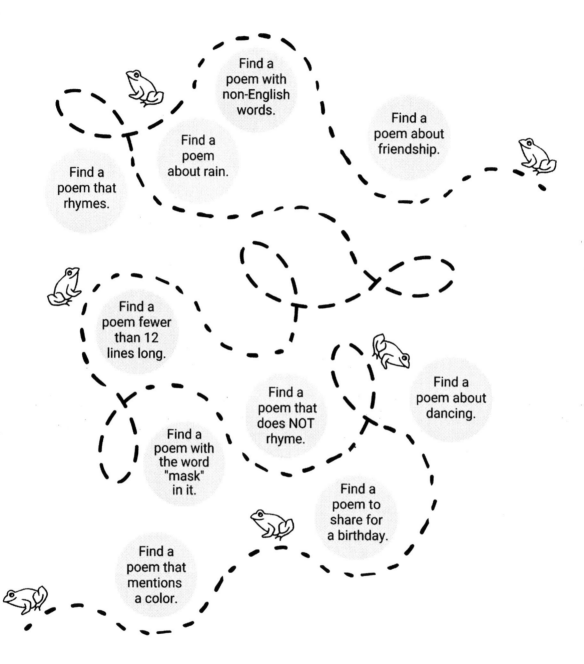

Find a poem with non-English words.

Find a poem about friendship.

Find a poem about rain.

Find a poem that rhymes.

Find a poem fewer than 12 lines long.

Find a poem that does NOT rhyme.

Find a poem about dancing.

Find a poem with the word "mask" in it.

Find a poem to share for a birthday.

Find a poem that mentions a color.

TIC TAC TOE

For 2-5 players: One person chooses poems to read, while others mark an image on their Tic Tac Toe card in a box that can fit that poem. Continue until someone fills a row and shouts TIC TAC TOE!!

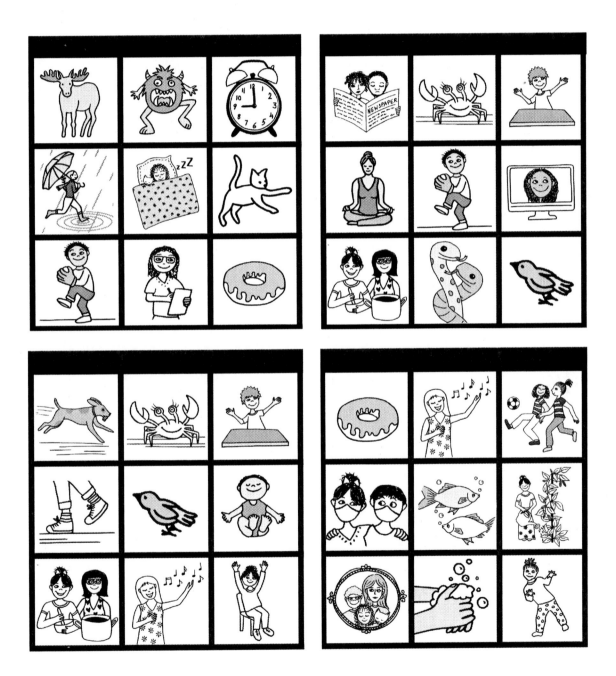

CREATE SOMETHING!

Write a poem of your own or draw a picture! Or BOTH!
Here are some words and images to get you thinking.

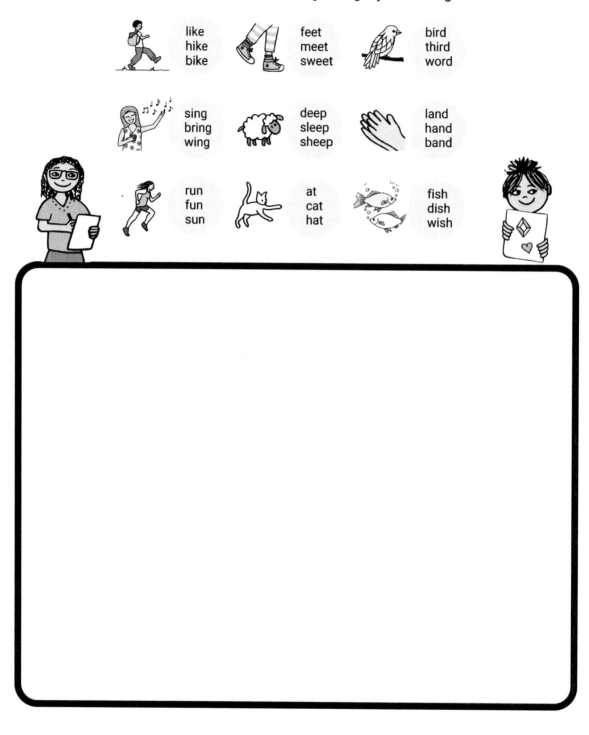

like
hike
bike

feet
meet
sweet

bird
third
word

sing
bring
wing

deep
sleep
sheep

land
hand
band

run
fun
sun

at
cat
hat

fish
dish
wish

POETRY MONTH CALENDAR

Celebrate National Poetry Month in April—or any month—with a poem a day. Make a note of the poem you share on each day or use these hints to find a fun poem. For example, you might choose a poem with a cat in it for Day 1, such as "Reach!" (p. 111). Use the subject index to find poems on specific topics that interest you.

Su	M	T	W	Th	F	Sa

POETRY CELEBRATIONS

For hundreds of years, people have been sharing poems for special occasions. Here are some ideas about special times for sharing a poem.

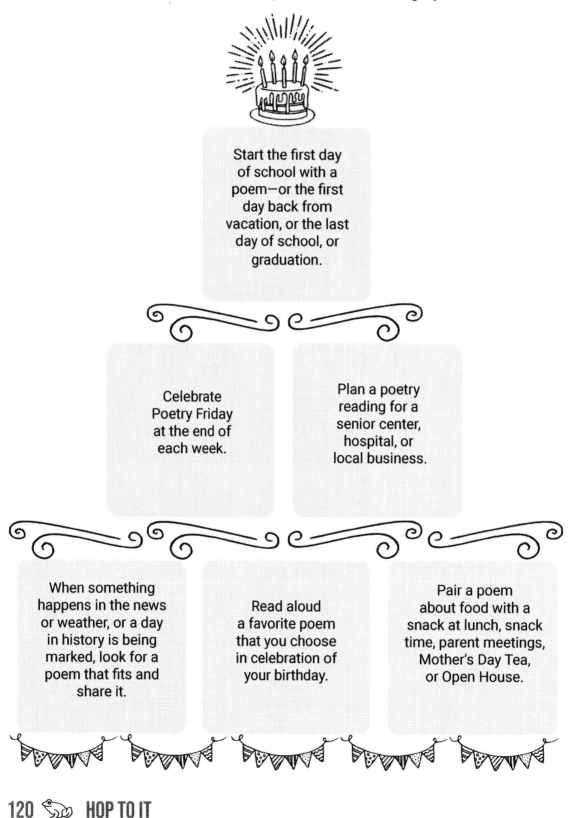

Start the first day of school with a poem—or the first day back from vacation, or the last day of school, or graduation.

Celebrate Poetry Friday at the end of each week.

Plan a poetry reading for a senior center, hospital, or local business.

When something happens in the news or weather, or a day in history is being marked, look for a poem that fits and share it.

Read aloud a favorite poem that you choose in celebration of your birthday.

Pair a poem about food with a snack at lunch, snack time, parent meetings, Mother's Day Tea, or Open House.

MIX IT UP

Once you get good at reading poems out loud, you might enjoy experimenting with other creative ways to make poetry come alive. Here are a few suggestions.

Use props and objects mentioned in the poem.

Cut out relevant paper or felt shapes while reading the poem.

Fold paper into origami shapes related to the poem.

Cook, mix, and bake along with the poem like a cooking show.

Perform poem using signing (American Sign Language).

Act out movements or emotions in the poem through pantomime.

Add simple dance moves to a poem with a lot of rhythm.

Flash a digital banner of a key poem line like a refrain.

Use simple movements like a hop or bounce for poems with a regular rhythm.

Create simple sound effects as the background for a poem reading.

Try chanting, hand claps, and/or jumping rope for strong rhythmic rhymes.

Add a musical soundtrack as the background for a poem performance.

Use video images to highlight key words and images in the poem.

Plan a *flash mob* reading of a favorite poem.

Try role playing (with hats or simple costumes) as a character in a poem that has a strong point of view.

Try using puppets or masks for a poem with characters.

ACT IT OUT

Here are some additional creative ideas for sharing a poem in dramatic ways that everyone will enjoy and remember.

Use **simple props** when reading a poem out loud. You can use a common object mentioned in the poem as your poetry prop and hold it up while reading aloud. Try making a video of yourself reading the poem using your prop and share it with a friend or send it to a relative. Using puppets can be fun too!

Add some **motions, movement, or pantomime** while you read a poem aloud to make a poem more fun. Act out the motions described in the poem while you read it or while a friend or family member reads it and you act it out. And if you know sign language, try signing the poem while a friend reads the poem aloud.

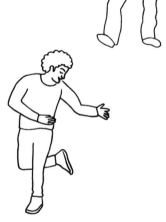

Use **music** in the background to create a special mood. A friend can play a musical instrument or you can find a recorded song or music. Think about whether you want to create a happy mood or a serious mood using the music and poem together.

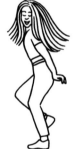

Translate your favorite poem into another language spoken in your community. You can work with a friend, someone in your family, a neighbor—or even just try working alone with Google Translate to see how your poem sounds in French, Chinese, Spanish, Arabic, or any other language.

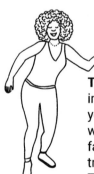

Use **sound effects** as a backdrop for your poem reading. A friend could make the sounds that go with the poem or you can find sounds and sound effects at places like SoundCloud.com. Think about making a podcast recording of the poem reading that you can share with others.

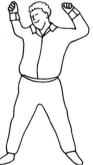

 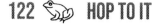

WAYS TO SHARE YOUR POEM

Once you try performing poems, you might enjoy experimenting with other creative ways to make poetry come alive. Here are a few suggestions.

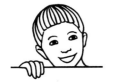

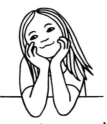

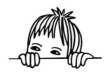

Copy or write your poem on a **postcard or letter** and mail it to a friend, someone in your family, or a neighbor. Or make a postcard with your poem and art on one side and the address on the other—and then mail it!

Find a **poetry pen-pal** and take turns passing your own original poems or some favorite poems found online back and forth with each other. Make a small book of the poems you've shared!

If you are able to text on a cell phone, try arranging a **text message** as a poem with line breaks or stanzas in different text bubbles. Or simply take a picture of your poem and send it with a text message.

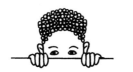

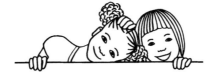

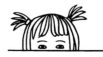

Make an audio recording or a video of yourself reading a poem out loud. Is there someone special you can send it to? Maybe you can send it to a relative you haven't seen for a while or a favorite teacher.

On **Poem in Your Pocket Day** in April, many people keep a poem or two in their pockets. Write poems on small cards to give away on that day and to keep in your pocket to share whenever you like.

Why not turn a blank card into a **greeting card** for a special occasion by writing your own poem on it and adding your own drawings? Make several cards now, so you'll have plenty to choose from when you need one.

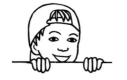

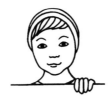

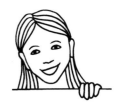

Make a poem into a **special gift.** Write it on a special or unusual piece of paper, add a drawing or painting or printed picture, and maybe even place it in a handmade frame as a small present for someone.

If you like using your computer to make art, there are many **digital tools** that you can use to create a collage or poster with your poem. Pick the images you like best and share them with your family.

Make your poem into a **3-D mobile.** Write each line of your poem on a different piece of heavy paper, and then tie string through each separate piece. Connect the pieces by hanging them on a stick or rod.

 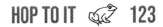

READ TOGETHER

It can be fun to read a poem aloud with a friend or your family.
Here are some different ways to do it.

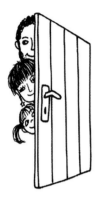

Poems that have a line or phrase that repeats more than once or that use number words like *two* or *ten* or *one hundred*, can be fun to read together. One person reads most of the poem aloud, but everyone joins in on the **repeated line** or phrase or number word.

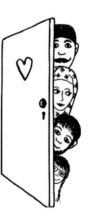

Echo reading is another way to read a poem aloud with a group when the poems have short lines. One person says each line of the poem, pausing at the end of each line so the rest of the group can repeat that line.

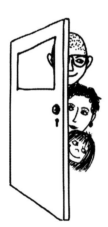

If there is **dialogue** in a poem, you can use it to create a dramatic reading too. A leader reads most of the poem aloud, and volunteers read the dialogue inside the quotation marks.

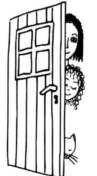

Invite guest readers to join you for poem readings to add variety. A coach, principal, grandparent, or athlete can each bring a different perspective, while readers who speak different languages can share poems from their languages.

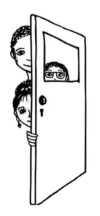

A poem that uses words in italics or bold can be perfect for **reading a poem in parts.** A leader reads most of the poem, while others read only the words in italics or bold. Take a moment to clarify whose line is whose, highlighting the text if that's helpful. Think about making a podcast recording of the reading, too.

 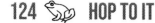

WEBSITES AND BLOGS TO KNOW

*There are several hundred websites and blogs that help us **find, share, and write poetry**.*
Here are a few of our favorites.

The Academy of American Poets
Poets.org
Promotes National Poetry Month, Poem-a-Day,
and offers hundreds of poems online.

Children's Poetry Archive
Childrens.PoetryArchive.org
Listen to hundreds of poems for young people
read aloud by the poets themselves.

No Water River: The Children's Poetry Place
NoWaterRiver.com
Watch videos of poets reading and talking
about their poetry.

Pinterest/PomeloBooks
Pinterest.com/PomeloBooks.com
Digital *postcards* featuring poems.

Poetry for Children by Sylvia Vardell
PoetryForChildren.Blogspot.com
Comprehensive resource with info about sharing
poetry.

Poetry Foundation Children's Page
Poetryfoundation.org/resources/children
Hundreds of poems and articles.

The Poetry Minute
PoetryMinute.org
Find a poem for every day, Monday through
Friday, from September to June.

There are many online resources that provide opportunities for young people to learn about how
*to **make a difference in the world**. You'll find links to many more resources at these websites.*

The Conscious Kid
TheConsciousKid.org
An education, research, and policy group
dedicated to equity and promoting healthy racial
identity development in youth.

The Malala Fund
Malala.org
This site encourages adults to donate time and
money to projects in honor of Malala Yousafzai,
but offers kids news and photos about the
program's impact on life for girls in countries
around the world.

A Mighty Girl
AMightyGirl.com
A resource site with recommendations of books
and more celebrating girls.

Raising Race Conscious Children
RaceConscious.org
A resource to support adults who want to talk
about race with young children.

Random Acts of Kindness Week
RandomActsofKindness.org
Look for opportunities to be a *RAKtivist* and
spread kindness in creative ways with notes,
tweets, gifts, and gestures.

There are many online resources that provide opportunities for young people to learn about how
*to **stay fit and healthy**. Again, here are just a handful to get you started.*

Be Active Kids
BeActiveKids.org
Interactive health program for adults who work
with children ages birth to five.

Kids Health
KidsHealth.org
This site strives to give families the tools
and confidence to make healthy choices.

Move Your Way
Health.gov/MoveYourWay
Tools, videos, and fact sheets that make
it easier to get a little more active.

**President's Council on Sports, Fitness
& Nutrition**
Fitness.gov
Promotes healthy and active lifestyles.

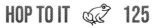

A MINI-GLOSSARY OF POETIC FORMS AND TECHNIQUES

All the poems in this book showcase poetic tools. In many cases, a single poem contains several features, but as a general rule we have chosen to highlight just one or two elements per poem. We feel that discussing too many techniques for a single poem can overwhelm students.

Alignment
Alignment is the way a poem is arranged with indentation and line breaks. Poets often play with alignment, especially when making revisions. A poet might decide to break a line right before or after a word to draw attention to it, or to place a word in a very short line to make it stand out. These poems contain interesting alignment choices:

Centered: "Chair Dancing" (p. 71).

Concrete poem (arranged in the shape of the subject of the poem): "This One" (p. 50).

Very short lines: "Clear, Cool Blue" (p. 86); "Waiting" (p. 68); "Wiggle Your Ears" (p. 69).

Alliteration
Alliteration involves the repetition of the same sound, particularly consonants, as the initial sound in a string of words. Other sound devices that are similar to alliteration are *consonance*, the repetition of the same consonant sound within words, and *assonance*, the repetition of the same vowel sound within words. You'll find examples of alliteration in: "Fit as a Fidget!" (p. 67); "Lockdown Freedom" (p. 43); "Reach!" (p. 111); "Same Friend, Different Size" (p. 20).

Capitalization and Font Choices
Poets often use *capitalization* and *font choices* (such as **bold** or *italics*) for style. Here are some examples of poems that use only lower case, italics, or capital letters to add to meaning and emphasize words. Note: when poets choose to use all lower case, they often also choose to omit punctuation, so some of these examples are repeated under **Punctuation**.

All lower case: "Everyday Use" (p. 60); "Footwork for Soccer Players Stuck Inside" (p. 80); "Wake the World" (p. 36).

Capitals at the start of each line: "2020" (p. 22); "Anyone Home?" (p. 91); "Soul Magic" (p. 109).

Capitalized words for emphasis: "Bones & Math" (p. 66); "City Song" (p. 52); "FREEZE" (p. 114).

Italics and capitals for emphasis: "Stand Up" (p. 57).

Free Verse
Free verse poems are poems that do not follow a set pattern or form and are usually irregular in line length. There can be some rhyming words scattered throughout a free verse poem (see **Internal Rhyme**), but there is no regular pattern of rhyme. See: "Look for Birds" (p. 29); "The Loudest of Hands" (p. 61); "One" (p. 107); "Umbrella" (p. 95); "Your Song" (p. 54).

 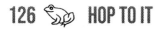

How-To Poem

A *how-to poem* is a form that is especially appealing to children. Usually it is a list poem, but it must also give specific directions on how to do something, as you'll find here: "A Poem for Tired Hands" (p. 64); "Banana Cake Beat" (p. 102); "Deskercise" (p. 72); "Hello, Friends" (p. 17); "Let's Dance" (p. 47); "On a Beach" (p. 85).

Imagery

Most poems contain images—words invoking or describing sensory perceptions and triggering one or more of the senses (sight, hearing, smell, touch, taste). One way to describe *imagery* to young children is to ask if a poem makes pictures in their minds. These poems contain particularly strong imagery: "Rabbit Dance" (p. 45); "What's Behind My Head?" (p. 21).

Internal Rhyme

The traditional form of *rhyme* that we are most familiar with is *end rhyme*, where rhyming words are placed at the ends of lines. We refer to *internal rhyme* when we find it within a line of poetry. When free verse poems contain any rhyme, it is often internal rhyme. See: "Follow Your Nose" (p. 34); "Now's Your Chance" (p. 38).

List Poem

A *list poem* lists words or phrases and often uses repetition (repeating either the exact words or repeating the structure of a line). Some list poems consist entirely of a list, but more commonly a list is found somewhere in the middle of the poem, with opening and closing lines that give the list some context: "#createachallenge" (p. 39); "'Do You Even Write on Your Birthday?'" (p. 100); "Rainbow Dance" (p. 96); "Staycation" (p. 32); "Stuck" (p. 41).

Lyrical Poem

Lyric (or *lyrical*) literally means *to be sung accompanied by the lyre*; a lyric (or lyrical) poem has come to mean a poem expressing the poet's emotions. Some poets use the term *in the lyrical voice* to describe first-person poems full of reflection: "Our Walk to School" (p. 28); "Say When" (p. 26); "Virtual Hoops" (p. 81).

Mask Poem

When the speaker in a poem is non-human and normally unable to talk, we can say that the poem is *in the voice of the mask*. Many mask poems are told from an animal's point of view: "I Stood on the Ceiling" (p. 103); "Pigeon Panache" (p. 44).

Metaphor and Simile

Metaphor is a figure of speech in which one thing or idea is represented by implicit comparison with another, while *simile* is an explicit comparison between two things or ideas, usually using *as* or *like*. Some metaphor poems never mention the *true* subject of the poem; for instance, in the poem "Look for Birds" (p. 29), one might say that birds could be a metaphor for change or good news—or they could just be birds.

Metaphor: "A Self-Trained Ninja" (p. 35); "At the Eye" (p. 93); "Zen Tree" (p. 84).

Simile: "Captain Toes" (p. 65); "In Nature" (p. 92); "Tae Kwon Do Punch" (p. 76); "Wave to Me from Across the Street!" (p. 19).

Meter and Rhythm

Meter is the pattern of stressed and unstressed syllables in verse that creates a distinctive *rhythm*. We often talk about meter in terms of types of metrical *feet* (such as iamb, anapest, trochee, and dactyl) and the number of them (three = trimeter, four = tetrameter, five = pentameter). Rhythm is the general term that describes a sense of movement or sound. One way to help children hear rhythm and meter is to tap or clap loudly when you read a stressed syllable, and to tap or clap softly when you hear an unstressed syllable. Note: unvarying *singsong* rhythm can be a problem in some poems, and poets sometimes choose to *break the rhythm* for emphasis. These poems have a particularly strong rhythm and/or a specific metrical pattern: "Ball Chant" (p. 78); "March!" (p. 58); "Pep Talk for a Couch Potato" (p. 113); "Tonight" (p. 104); "When I Move" (p. 112); "Zoom Doom" (p. 42).

Narrative Poem

A *narrative* poem tells a story, usually from the point of view of a third-person narrator: "All Tied, Bases Loaded" (p. 79); "Sato Dog and Little Blue Crab" (p. 88).

Onomatopoeia

Onomatopoeia is the term for words that capture the sounds they describe, such as many animal sounds; loud, startling sounds; and weather sounds: "Be the Beat!" (p. 49); "Exercising My Voice" (p. 55); "Monsters Don't Dance" (p. 46).

Personification

Personification describes non-human things in human terms: "A Poem for When Things Get a Little Too Serious" (p. 30); "Any Weather" (p. 94). Personification is usually present in mask poems and *apostrophe* poems.

Poem of Address (or Apostrophe Poem)

In a *poem of address*, the poet speaks directly to a subject, often using the word *you*. When poets speak to someone or something who cannot possibly answer, such as an idea, inanimate object, or historical figure, then we can say they are using *apostrophe*: "Calling All Kids" (p. 108); "No Matter What" (p. 105); "Rise Up Tall" (p. 83); "Walking" (p. 59).

Punctuation

Poets often use *punctuation* for style. Here are some examples of poems that use punctuation in an interesting way (or omit it completely).

Ellipses: "The Great Indoors" (p. 33); "Superhero" (p. 110).

One long sentence: "Changing Times" (p. 27).

No punctuation: "A New Day" (p. 37); "Everyday Use" (p. 60); "Footwork for Soccer Players Stuck Inside" (p. 80).

Parentheses: "Trail Ready" (p. 82).

Question Poem

A *question poem* uses questions as an important element: "Can You Wiggle Like a Worm?" (p. 90); "I Smile with My Eyes" (p. 25); "Walk One Mile" (p. 18).

 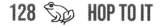

Repetition

Repetition involves repeating sounds, words, phrases, or sentence structures again and again in a poem, usually for musical effect or enhanced meaning: "Can I Please Have a Calendar?" (p. 40); "Heartbeat" (p. 53); "My Desk Is a Race Car" (p. 73); "Warmup Chant" (p. 74); "When I Feel Scared" (p. 98); "You Can Do It Right Now" (p. 56); "You Can't Catch Me" (p. 89).

Rhyme

Rhyme describes the matching of syllable sounds and is usually found at the ends of lines of verse (see **Internal Rhyme** for an exception). Note: some poets deliberately avoid using exact rhyme, preferring instead to rely on assonance, consonance, and words that almost rhyme (variations are called near rhyme, off rhyme, sight rhyme, and slant rhyme). Rhyme is often used in poems arranged in stanzas called *couplets*, *tercets*, and *quatrains* (see more under **Stanza**). You'll find many outstanding examples of rhyme throughout this book, but look to these poems for some distinctive rhyming words or rhyme *schemes* (patterns): "I Smile with My Eyes" (p. 25); "Micro Monster" (p. 23); "The P.E. Instructor Teaches a Class of Young Snakes" (p. 77).

Stanza

A *stanza* is a group of lines presented together without any line spaces.

Single stanza

Many free verse poems are presented as a single block of text, but sometimes poems with a regular pattern of end rhyme are also arranged into a single stanza: "Click! Clack! Jumping Jack!" (p. 75); "Music in My Town" (p. 51); "Tonight" (p. 104).

Couplet

A two-line stanza: "Hands Say 'Great Job'" (p. 62); "Hand Washing Song" (p. 63); "Me and the Beach Creatures" (p. 87); "Raindrops and Words" (p. 97).

Tercet

A three-line stanza: "Hop to It" (p. 15); "Mental Floss" (p. 70).

Quatrain

A four-line stanza: "Cumpleaños imaginario / A Make-Believe Birthday" (p. 101); "Feel the Beat" (p. 48); "Masks for All!" (p. 24); "Micro Monster" (p. 23); "The Artist" (p. 99).

Tanka (and Haiku)

A *tanka* is an ancient Japanese poetic form that usually consists of five lines with syllable counts of 5-7-5-7-7. It is not necessary to follow a strict syllable count and, in fact, poets devoted to tanka and haiku often ignore syllable counts. Unlike haiku—more than just a 5-7-5 syllabic form, but rather a poem that focuses our attention on nature and seasons—tanka do not involve nature and ordinarily feature a lyrical element focusing on human relationships: "When I Close My Eyes" (p. 106).

Wordplay

Poets love to play with words by using unusual words, inventing new words (often to create puns), and twisting phrases, especially for humor. See: "Carelessly Hairless" (p. 31); "The P.E. Instructor Teaches a Class of Young Snakes" (p. 77); "Ways to Say Hello" (p. 16).

 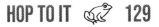

PICTURE BOOK PAIRINGS FOR EVERY POEM

Alexander, Kwame. 2019. *How to Read a Book*. HarperCollins. (p. 12)

Arnold, Tedd. 2006. *Hi! Fly Guy*. Cartwheel Books. (p. 103)

Ashman, Linda. 2020. *When the Storm Comes*. Nancy Paulsen Books. (p. 94)

Baicker, Karen. 2010. *I Can Do It Too!* Chronicle. (p. 111)

Barnes, Derrick. 2020. *I Am Every Good Thing*. Nancy Paulsen Books. (p. 60)

Bates, Amy June and Bates, Juniper. 2018. *The Big Umbrella*. Simon & Schuster. (p. 95)

Baumgarten, Bret and Otoshi, Kathryn. 2015. *Beautiful Hands*. Blue Dot. (p. 62)

Beaty, Andrea. 2019. *Sofia Valdez, Future Prez*. Abrams. (p. 112)

Ben-Barak, Idan. 2018. *Do Not Lick This Book*. Roaring Brook. (p. 22)

Biebow, Natascha. 2019. *The Crayon Man*. Houghton Mifflin Harcourt. (p. 96)

Bishop, Nic. 2012. *Snakes*. Scholastic. (p. 77)

Bolling, Valerie. 2020. *Let's Dance*. Boyds Mills Press. (p. 47)

Brisson, Pat. 2018. *Before We Eat*. Tilbury House. (p. 105)

Bruchac, Joseph and Bruchac, James. 2012. *Rabbit's Snow Dance*. Dial. (p. 45)

Burningham, John. 2014. *The Way to the Zoo*. Candlewick. (p. 43)

Byers, Grace. 2018. *I Am Enough*. Balzer + Bray. (p. 108)

Chen, Eva. 2018. *Juno Valentine and the Magical Shoes*. Feiwel & Friends. (p. 18)

Chin, Jason. 2015. *Redwoods*. Square Fish. (p. 83)

Clark-Robinson, Monica. 2018. *Let the Children March*. Houghton Mifflin Harcourt. (p. 58)

Cline-Ransome, Lesa. 2017. *Germs*. Holt. (p. 24)

Coffelt, Nancy. 2011. *Fred Stays with Me!* Little, Brown. (p. 34)

Cooper, Elisha. 2006. *Beach*. Orchard. (p. 85)

Cooper, Elisha. 2019. *River*. Orchard. (p. 92)

Cooper, Jenny. 2017. *Do Your Ears Hang Low?* Sterling. (p. 69)

Craig, Lindsey. 2010. *Dancing Feet!* Knopf. (p. 67)

Crockett-Corson, Kim. 2017. *My Good Morning*. Clavis. (p. 37)

Cronin, Doreen. 2005. *Wiggle*. Atheneum. (p. 65)

Davies, Jacqueline. 2007. *The House Takes a Vacation*. Two Lions. (p. 30)

Davis, Katie. 2001. *Who Hops?* Houghton Mifflin Harcourt. (p. 10)

Detlefsen, Lisl H. 2019. *1, 2, 3, Jump!* Roaring Brook. (p. 86)

Doerrfeld, Cori. 2018. *The Rabbit Listened*. Dial. (p. 106)

Dyckman, Ame. 2012. *Boy + Bot*. Knopf. (p. 26)

Egan, Tim. 2007. *The Pink Refrigerator*. Houghton Mifflin Harcourt. (p. 39)

Engle, Margarita. 2015. *Drum Dream Girl*. Houghton Mifflin Harcourt. (p. 49)

Farrell, Alison. 2019. *The Hike*. Chronicle. (p. 82)

Flood, Nancy Bo. 2020. *I Will Dance*. Atheneum. (p. 71)

Grey, Mini. 2012. *Traction Man Is Here*. Dragonfly Books. (p. 110)

Harrington, Janice N. 2019. *Buzzing with Questions*. Calkins Creek. (p. 89)

Haughton, Chris. 2020. *Don't Worry, Little Crab*. Chronicle. (p. 88)

Henderson, Leah. 2020. *Mamie on the Mound*. Capstone. (p. 79)

Henkes, Kevin. 2009. *Birds*. Greenwillow. (p. 29)

Henkes, Kevin. 2015. *Waiting*. Greenwillow. (p. 68)

Hubbard, Rita Lorraine. 2020. *The Oldest Student*. Schwartz & Wade. (p. 13)

Jenkins, Steve. 2010. *Bones*. Scholastic. (p. 66)

Jenkins, Steve. 2009. *Never Smile at a Monkey*. Houghton Mifflin Harcourt. (p. 25)

John, Jory. 2020. *The Couch Potato*. HarperCollins. (p. 113)

Joy, Angela. 2020. *Black Is a Rainbow Color*. Roaring Brook. (p. 109)

Jules, Jacqueline. 2020. *Tag Your Dreams*. Albert Whitman. (p. 114)

Krall, Dan. 2020. *Sick Simon*. Simon & Schuster. (p. 41)

Krishnaswami, Uma. 2018. *Book Uncle and Me*. Groundwood. (p. 11)

Krishnaswami, Uma. 2008. *The Happiest Tree*. Lee & Low. (p. 84)

Krosoczka, Jarrett K. 2005. *Punk Farm*. Knopf. (p. 52)

Levine, Arthur A. 2011. *Monday Is One Day*. Scholastic. (p. 40)

Littlejohn, James. 2018. *B Is for Baller*. Triumph Books. (p. 81)

Mabbit, Will. 2019. *I Can Only Draw Worms*. Penguin. (p. 90)

Maillard, Kevin Noble. 2019. *Fry Bread*. Roaring Brook. (p. 102)

Mann, Jennifer K. 2020. *The Camping Trip*. Candlewick. (p. 33)

Marley, Bob. 2019. *Get Up, Stand Up*. Chronicle. (p. 57)

McDaniel, Breanna J. 2019. *Hands Up!* Dial. (p. 61)

McElligott, Matthew. 2010. *Even Monsters Need Haircuts*. Bloomsbury. (p. 31)

Metcalf, Lindsay H. et al. (Eds.). 2020. *No Voice Too Small*. Charlesbridge. (p. 55)

Miller, Pat Zietlow. 2019. *When You Are Brave*. Little, Brown. (p. 98)

Mora, Oge. 2019. *Saturday*. Little, Brown. (p. 28)

Napoli, Donna Jo. 2014. *Hands & Hearts*. Abrams. (p. 17)

Newman, Jeff. 2011. *Hand Book*. Simon & Schuster. (p. 64)

Ode, Eric. 2018. *Sea Star Wishes*. Little Bigfoot. (p. 87)

O'Leary, Sara. 2016. *A Family Is a Family Is a Family*. Groundwood. (p. 27)

Olson, Jennifer Gray. 2015. *Ninja Bunny*. Knopf. (p. 35)

Parr, Todd. 2020. *The Birthday Book*. Little, Brown. (p. 101)

Paul, Baptiste and Paul, Miranda. 2019. *I Am Farmer*. Millbrook. (p. 104)

Penfold, Alexandra. 2018. *All Are Welcome*. Knopf. (p. 59)

Piercy, Helen. 2013. *Animation Studio*. Candlewick. (p. 21)

Pinkney, Andrea Davis. 2010. *Sit-In*. Little, Brown. (p. 56)

Raschka, Chris. 2011. *A Ball for Daisy*. Schwartz & Wade. (p. 78)

Rechler, Lindsay. 2020. *Good Morning Zoom*. Philomel. (p. 42)

Reynolds, Peter H. *The Word Collector*. Orchard. (p. 54)

Rockwell, Lizzy. 2004. *The Busy Body Book*. Crown. (p. 75)

Ruurs, Margriet. 2004. *When We Go Camping*. Tundra. (p. 32)

Santat, Dan. 2014. *The Adventures of Beekle*. Little, Brown. (p. 20)

Say, Allen. 2003. *Emma's Rug*. Houghton Mifflin Harcourt. (p. 99)

Schwartz, Corey Rosen. 2014. *Ninja Red Riding Hood*. Crown. (p. 76)

Sendak, Maurice. 1963. *Where the Wild Things Are*. HarperCollins. (p. 46)

Shaw, Charles. 1988. *It Looked Like Spilt Milk*. HarperCollins. (p. 97)

Singer, Marilyn. 2017. *Feel the Beat*. Dial. (p. 70)

Singh, Simran Jeet. 2020. *Fauja Singh Keeps Going*. Kokila. (p. 74)

Smith, Cynthia Leitich. 2000. *Jingle Dancer*. HarperCollins. (p. 48)

Snider, Grant. 2020. *What Sound Is Morning?* Chronicle. (p. 36)

Spires, Ashley. 2017. *The Thing Lou Couldn't Do*. Kids Can Press. (p. 38)

Stead, Philip C. 2010. *A Sick Day for Amos McGee*. Roaring Brook. (p. 23)

Steinglass, Elizabeth. 2019. *Soccerverse*. Wordsong/Boyds Mills. (p. 80)

Stutson, Caroline. 2010. *Cats' Night Out*. Paula Wiseman Books. (p. 51)

Thompson, Lauren. 2012. *Hop, Hop, Jump!* Margaret K. McElderry Books. (p. 15)

Turk, Evan. 2018. *Heartbeat*. Atheneum. (p. 53)

Van Dusen, Chris. 2019. *If I Built a School*. Dial. (p. 73)

Verdick, Elizabeth. 2011. *Germs Are Not for Sharing*. Free Spirit. (p. 63)

Weatherford, Carole Boston. 2019. *The Roots of Rap*. little bee books. (p. 50)

Wenzel, Brendan. 2019. *A Stone Sat Still*. Chronicle. (p. 91)

Wenzel, Brendan. 2018. *Hello Hello*. Chronicle. (p. 16)

Willems, Mo. 2003. *Don't Let the Pigeon Drive the Bus*. Hyperion. (p. 44)

Wong, Janet. 2007. *Twist*. Margaret K. McElderry Books. (p. 72)

Wong, Janet. 2002. *You Have to Write*. Margaret K. McElderry Books. (p. 100)

Woodson, Jacqueline. 2018. *The Day You Begin*. Nancy Paulsen Books. (p. 107)

Woodson, Jacqueline. 2001. *The Other Side*. Putnam. (p. 19)

Yolen, Jane and Stemple, Heidi E.Y. 2020. *I Am the Storm*. Penguin. (p. 93)

POETRY BOOKS ABOUT SOCIAL JUSTICE

In these books, poets write about social justice issues and about people who have fought for equality and civil rights.

Ada, Alma Flor and Campoy, Isabel F. 2013. *Yes! We Are Latinos*. Charlesbridge.

Argueta, Jorge. 2016. *Somos como las nubes / We Are Like the Clouds*. Groundwood.

Bernier-Grand, Carmen T. 2004. *César: Sí, se puede! Yes, We Can!* Marshall Cavendish.

Boyce, Jo Ann Allen and Levy, Debbie. 2018. *This Promise of Change*. Harper.

Browne, Mahogany L. 2020. *Woke*. Roaring Brook Press.

Cheng, Andrea. 2013. *Etched in Clay*. Lee & Low.

Clark-Robinson, Monica. 2018. *Let the Children March*. Houghton Mifflin Harcourt.

Corcoran, Jill (Ed.). 2012. *Dare to Dream . . . Change the World*. Kane Miller.

Elliott, Zetta. 2019. *Say Her Name*. Disney-Hyperion.

Engle, Margarita. 2006. *The Poet Slave of Cuba*. Henry Holt.

Engle, Margarita. 2010. *The Firefly Letters*. Henry Holt.

Engle, Margarita. 2013. *The Lightning Dreamer*. Houghton Mifflin Harcourt.

Engle, Margarita. 2014. *Silver People*. Houghton Mifflin Harcourt.

Hudson, Wade and Hudson, Cheryl Willis. 2018. *We Rise, We Resist, We Raise Our Voices*. Crown.

Hughes, Langston. 2009. *My People*. Ill. by Charles R. Smith, Jr. Simon & Schuster.

Johnson, Maureen (Ed.). 2018. *How I Resist*. Wednesday Books.

Latham, Irene and Waters, Charles. 2017. *Can I Touch Your Hair?* Millbrook Press.

Lewis, J. Patrick and Lyon, George Ella. 2014. *Voices from the March*. Wordsong/Boyds Mills.

Lewis, J. Patrick. 2013. *When Thunder Comes*. Chronicle.

Lyon, George Ella. 2020. *Voices of Justice*. Holt.

Metcalf, Lindsay; Dawson, Keila; and Bradley, Jeanette (Eds.). 2020. *No Voice Too Small*. Charlesbridge.

Myers, Walter Dean. 2011. *We Are America*. HarperCollins.

Nelson, Marilyn. 2009. *Sweethearts of Rhythm*. Dial.

Otheguy, Emma. 2017. *Martí's Song for Freedom*. Lee & Low.

Rappaport, Doreen. 2006. *Nobody Gonna Turn Me 'Round*. Candlewick.

Shovan, Laura. 2016. *The Last Fifth Grade of Emerson Elementary*. Random House.

Weatherford, Carole Boston. 2002. *Remember the Bridge*. Philomel.

Weatherford, Carole Boston. 2007. *Birmingham, 1963*. Wordsong/Boyds Mills.

Weatherford, Carole Boston. 2015. *Voice of Freedom*. Candlewick.

Wong, Janet. 2012. *Declaration of Interdependence*. PoetrySuitcase.

POETRY BOOKS ABOUT SPORTS, DANCE, AND MOVEMENT

Sports and poetry may seem like an unlikely combination, but it has ancient roots with poems recited at sporting events such as victory odes at the earliest Olympics. Plus these poems capture the thrill of movement, the rewards of teamwork, and the release of physical exercise and can be performed with gestures, pantomime, movement, and audience cheers.

Alexander, Kwame. 2014. *The Crossover*. Houghton Mifflin Harcourt.

Brown, Marc. 2013. *Marc Brown's Playtime Rhymes*. Little, Brown.

Burg, Ann. 2009. *All the Broken Pieces*. Scholastic.

Dotlich, Rebecca Kai. 2004. *Over in the Pink House*. Wordsong/Boyds Mills.

Fehler, Gene. 2009. *Change-up*. Clarion.

Fitch, Sheree. 2019. *Toes in My Nose*. Nimbus Publishing.

Flood, Nancy Bo. 2013. *Cowboy Up! Ride the Navajo Rodeo*. Wordsong/Boyds Mills.

Florian, Douglas. 2012. *Poem Runs*. Houghton Mifflin Harcourt.

Franco, Betsy. 2009. *Messing Around the Monkey Bars*. Candlewick.

Hopkins, Lee Bennett (Ed.). 1999. *Sports! Sports! Sports!* HarperCollins.

Hoyte, Carol-Ann and Roemer, Heidi Bee (Eds.). 2012. *And the Crowd Goes Wild!* Friesens Press.

Jules, Jacqueline. 2020. *Tag Your Dreams*. Albert Whitman.

Katz, Alan. 2009. *Going, Going, Gone! And Other Silly Dilly Sports Songs*. Simon & Schuster.

Landry, Leo. 2019. *Home Run, Touchdown, Basket, Goal!* Henry Holt.

Low, Alice. 2009. *The Fastest Game on Two Feet*. Holiday House.

Lowe, Ayana. 2008. *Come and Play*. Bloomsbury.

Maddox, Marjorie. 2009. *Rules of the Game*. Wordsong/Boyds Mills.

McKissack, Patricia. 2017. *Let's Clap, Jump, Sing and Shout*. Random House/Schwartz & Wade.

Prelutsky, Jack. 2007. *Good Sports*. Knopf.

Shiefman, Vicky. 2019. *Who Has Wiggle-Waggle Toes?* Holiday House.

Silberg, Jackie and Schiller, Pam (Eds.). 2002. *The Complete Book of Rhymes*. Gryphon House.

Singer, Marilyn. 2011. *A Stick Is an Excellent Thing*. Clarion.

Singer, Marilyn. 2017. *Feel the Beat*. Dial.

Smith, Charles R., Jr. 2004. *Diamond Life*. Orchard.

Steinglass, Elizabeth. 2019. *Soccerverse*. Boyds Mills/Wordsong.

Stoop, Naoko. 2016. *Sing with Me! Action Songs Every Child Should Know*. Henry Holt.

Weisburd, Stefi. 2008. *Barefoot*. Wordsong/Boyds Mills.

Wong, Janet. 2007. *Twist*. Margaret K. McElderry Books.

SUBJECT INDEX

TITLE INDEX

 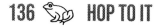

POET INDEX

POEM CREDITS

Each of the poems listed below is used with the permission of the author, with all rights reserved. To request reprint rights, please write us at info@pomelobooks.com, and we will put you in touch with the poets or their agents.

Alma Flor Ada: "A Make-Believe Birthday / Cumpleaños imaginario"; © 2020 by Alma Flor Ada.

Kathryn Apel: "Fit as a Fidget!"; © 2020 by Kathryn Apel.

Rebecca Balcárcel: "Any Weather," "Reach!"; © 2020 by Rebecca Balcárcel.

Ibtisam Barakat: "Raindrops and Words"; © 2020 by Ibtisam Barakat.

Michelle Heidenrich Barnes: "All Tied, Bases Loaded"; © 2020 by Michelle Heidenrich Barnes.

Doraine Bennett: "Your Song"; © 2020 by Doraine Bennett.

Carmen T. Bernier-Grand: "Sato Dog and Little Blue Crab"; © 2020 by Carmen T. Bernier-Grand.

Robyn Hood Black: "Trail Ready"; © 2020 by Robyn Hood Black.

Susan Blackaby: "Me and the Beach Creatures"; © 2020 by Susan Blackaby.

David Bowles: "Music in My Town"; © 2020 by David Bowles.

Jay Brazeau: "Wiggle Your Ears!"; © 2020 by Jay Brazeau.

Joseph Bruchac: "Rabbit Dance"; © 2020 by Joseph Bruchac.

Stephanie Calmenson: "Feel the Beat"; © 2020 by Stephanie Calmenson.

F. Isabel Campoy: "En la naturaleza / In Nature"; © 2020 by F. Isabel Campoy.

Rose Cappelli: "Can You Wiggle Like a Worm?"; © 2020 by Rose Cappelli.

Yangsook Choi: "A Self-Trained Ninja," "Tae Kwon Do Punch"; © 2020 by Yangsook Choi.

Lesa Cline-Ransome: "A New Day"; © 2020 by Lesa Cline-Ransome.

Natalee Creech: "A Poem for Tired Hands"; © 2020 by Natalee Creech

Ed DeCaria: "Warmup Chant"; © 2020 by Ed DeCaria.

Kristy Dempsey: "#createachallenge," "What's Behind My Head?"; © 2020 by Kristy Dempsey.

Linda Dryfhout: "Let's Dance"; © 2020 by Linda Dryfhout.

Alice Faye Duncan: "Soul Magic"; © 2020 by Alice Faye Duncan.

Zetta Elliott: "Everyday Use"; © 2020 by Zetta Elliott.

Margarita Engle: "Follow Your Nose"; © 2020 by Margarita Engle.

Janet Clare Fagal: "Calling All Kids"; © 2020 by Janet Clare Fagal.

Carrie Finison: "Pigeon Panache"; © 2020 by Carrie Finison.

Nancy Bo Flood: "Anyone Home?"; © 2020 by Nancy Bo Flood.

Catherine Flynn: "Mental Floss"; © 2020 by Catherine Flynn.

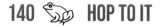

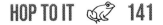

ABOUT THE CREATORS

Sylvia Vardell is Professor in the School of Library and Information Studies at Texas Woman's University and teaches graduate courses in children's and young adult literature. Vardell has published extensively, including five books on literature for children as well as over 25 book chapters and 100 journal articles. Her current work focuses on poetry for children, including a regular blog, PoetryforChildren.Blogspot.com. Vardell has served as a member or chair of several national award committees, including the NCTE Award for Poetry, the ALA Legacy Award, and the Odyssey, Sibert, and Caldecott award committees, among others. She has conducted over 150 presentations at state, regional, national, and international conferences. She taught at the University of Zimbabwe in Africa as a Fulbright scholar and was a recipient of the Scholastic Library Publishing Award. Learn more about her at **SylviaVardell.com**.

What gets Sylvia up and moving? Walking all over her neighborhood, taking trips and walking in brand new places, and walking for miles at Star Wars conventions.

Janet Wong is a graduate of Yale Law School and a former lawyer who switched careers to become a children's author. Her dramatic career change has been featured on *The Oprah Winfrey Show*, CNN's *Paula Zahn Show*, and *Radical Sabbatical*. She is the author of more than 30 books for children and teens on a wide variety of subjects, including writing and revision (*You Have to Write*), diversity and community (*Apple Pie 4th of July*), peer pressure (*Me and Rolly Maloo*), chess (*Alex and the Wednesday Chess Club*), and yoga (*Twist: Yoga Poems*). A frequent featured speaker at literacy conferences, Wong has served as a member of several national committees, including the NCTE Poetry Committee and the ILA Notable Books for a Global Society committee. Her current focus is encouraging children to publish their own writing using affordable new technologies. Learn more about her at **JanetWong.com**.

The activities that get Janet up and moving are walking with her dog, gardening, and doing yoga.

Franzi Paetzold is a freelance illustrator from Germany. As a globetrotter and former social worker, she has spent much of her life traveling the world, studying and working abroad. In between work and plane rides, she started publishing her drawings online and taking on small assignments. She now illustrates full time, and lives with a friend and two friendly cats in Berlin. Her illustrations can be found at **FranziDraws.com**.

What gets Franzi up and moving? Going for walks along the nearby river, capoeira, swimming, and (of course) traveling.

ABOUT POMELO BOOKS

Pomelo Books was created in 2012 with the goal of making it easy for teachers and librarians to share poetry. While our early books in *The Poetry Friday Anthology*™ series focused on teaching poetry as part of the language arts standards, our later books addressed the need for poems that could be shared across the curriculum, such as poems about science, technology, engineering, math, and social studies—as well as social-emotional learning, especially with *GREAT MORNING! Poems for School Leaders to Read Aloud*. We expanded our focus again with the *Poetry Friday Power Book* series of interactive journals that provide a bridge between reading and writing, and that are used by many young readers and writers for supplemental learning at home.

Our emphasis in all our books has been to highlight diversity and inclusion through a wide variety of *21st-century* topics and a multitude of original and distinctive voices, both established and new.

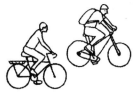

Life is like riding a bicycle.
To keep your balance,
you must keep moving.
ALBERT EINSTEIN

GET "POETRY PLUS!" WITH POMELO BOOKS

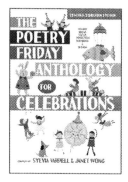

The Poetry Friday Anthology for Celebrations
ILA 2016 Notable Books for a Global Society

Teacher/Librarian Edition (K-8)
Each of the 156 poems has a *Take 5!* mini-lesson with picture book pairings. Matrixes highlight social studies and language arts connections.

Student Edition (K-8)
This companion volume for children features illustrations (no mini-lessons). Listen to 35 poems in Spanish & English—FREE at SoundCloud.com!

"A bubbly and educational bilingual poetry anthology for children." —*Kirkus*

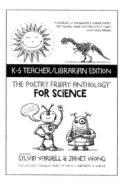

The Poetry Friday Anthology for Science
NSTA Recommends
Featured on ScienceFriday.com + in a monthly column in *Science & Children*
You'll find 250+ poems on science, technology, engineering, and math.

K-5 Teacher/Librarian Edition (K-5)
Each poem is accompanied by a *Take 5!* mini-lesson with both language arts and science-themed teaching tips.

Student Edition (K-8)
The Poetry of Science is an illustrated companion volume for children that is organized by topic and features illustrations (no mini-lessons).

"A treasury of the greatest science poetry for children ever written, with a twist" —**NSTA Recommends**

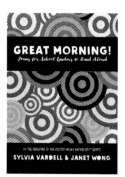

GREAT MORNING! Poems for School Leaders to Read Aloud

A CBC Hot Off the Press Selection
75 poems for morning announcements—or for the start of class, or just to insert a "brain break" when you need it!

Each of these poems has a ready-to-read "Did You Know?" introduction that you can read aloud, as well as a "Follow Up" for closure and a "Connect" piece for a text-to-text connection later in the week.

FOR AT-HOME LEARNING:
THE POETRY FRIDAY POWER BOOK SERIES

You Just Wait: A Poetry Friday Power Book
(Grades 5 and up)
An NCTE Poetry Notable

This interactive story in poems and writing journal centers around identity, diversity, movies, and sports (soccer and basketball). Extensive back matter resources for readers and writers.

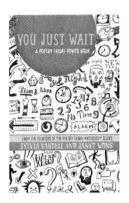

> **"This delightful collection . . . makes both reading and writing poetry personal and accessible to even the most resistant."**
> —*School Library Journal*

Here We Go: A Poetry Friday Power Book
(Grades 3 and up)
An NCTE Poetry Notable
An NNSTOY Social Justice Book

This interactive story inspires kids with themes of diversity and social activism (organizing a walkathon, canned food drive, and school garden). Extensive back matter resources for young writers and kids who want to change the world.

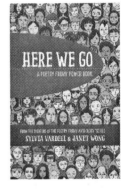

> **"Filled with poems by a variety of award-winning poets, this engaging resource invites readers to 'power up' and explore the world of poetry."**—*Literacy Daily*

Pet Crazy: A Poetry Friday Power Book
(Grades K-4)
A CBC Hot Off the Press selection

This interactive story—with Hidden Language Skills that engage kids in "playing" with punctuation, spelling, and other basics—features three characters who love spending time with animals. Extensive back matter features resources for helping young people perform, read, write, and try to publish poetry.

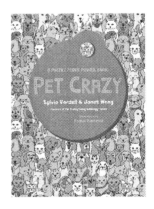

> **"An enthusiastic invitation for kids to celebrate their animal friends through poetry composition."**—*Kirkus*

FIND FREE SAMPLE POEMS AT PINTEREST.COM/POMELOBOOKS
FIND FREE POEM VIDEOS AT VIMEO.COM/POMELOBOOKS